'A non-faddy diet that offers incredible health benefits and weight loss. Aidan and Glen show how everyone can reap the benefits of the Sirtfood Diet through eating delicious food. I'm a huge fan!'
Lorraine Pascale, BBC TV chef and food writer

'A revelation to my diet. With the help of Aidan and Glen, introducing Sirtfoods has allowed me to attain a body composition and well-being previously unimaginable.'
David Haye, Champion heavyweight boxer

'People keep asking me my secret to looking great. The answer is Aidan and Glen's Sirtfood Diet. Since following it, I feel unstoppable.'
Jodie Kidd, Model and TV personality

'Working with Aidan and Glen has revolutionised my nutritional approach beyond anything I have experienced in the past. Their knowledge and Sirtfood Diet is unrivalled, and was key for getting me into top shape and feeling and performing at my best for the 2015 Rugby World Cup.'
James Haskell, International England Rugby star

'Following Aidan and Glen's Sirtfood Diet was incredible; my body fat just melted away, I was sharper and had heaps more energy than before.'
Anthony Ogogo, 2015 Strictly Come Dancing star and professional boxer

'I'm healthier, more alert and in top physical condition. Sirtfoods are key to me reaching new peaks in performance to face the upcoming challenges in making British America's Cup history.'
Sir Ben Ainslie, Four-times Olympic gold medallist

'Thank you! My husband is looking extra hot.'

The wife of one of the Sirtfood Diet participants after he lost 7lb 8oz (3.4kg) in 7 days

'The initial day was tough, but after that I felt my energy levels surge and I slept better. I think one challenging day is worth a lifetime of health.'

James M., lost 7lb 4oz (3.3kg) in 7 days

'The diet got me in the shape of my life just in time for my wedding day.'

Jadis T., lost over 6lb (2.7kg) including gaining 2lb (900g) of muscle in 7 days

'It might just be a lifesaver.'

David C., lost over 24lb (11kg) and reversed metabolic disease in 6 months

Aidan Goggins

Driven by his quest to cure his own rare autoimmune disease, Aidan is, unusually, both a pharmacist and nutritionist. It is this unique mix that has led to Aidan becoming one of Europe's most sought-after health experts, with clients ranging from doctors to celebrity personalities. A huge fitness enthusiast, he specialises in sports nutrition and his dietary expertise underpins the success of many champion professional athletes. Aidan is a prominent health commentator in the media as well as an award-winning writer.

Glen Matten

With a master's degree in nutritional medicine and a predilection for good food, Glen is a nutrition nerd and full-on foodie in equal measures. Glen has run successful clinics across the UK for over a decade and his clients include a number of professional athletes and celebrities. He is an award-winning author who makes frequent forays into the media.

the
sirt
food diet

AIDAN GOGGINS & GLEN MATTEN

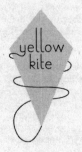

First published in Great Britain in 2016 by Yellow Kite
An imprint of Hodder & Stoughton
An Hachette UK company

9

A CIP catalogue record for this title is
available from the British Library

Trade Paperback ISBN 978 1 473 62678 2
eBook ISBN 9781473626805

Typeset in Sabon MT by Palimpsest Book Production Limited,
Falkirk, Stirlingshire
Printed and bound by CPI Group (UK) Ltd, Croydon, CR0 4YY

The advice herein is not intended to replace the services of trained health professionals,
or be a substitute for medical advice. You are advised to consult with your health
care professional with regards to matters relating to your health, and in particular
regarding matters that may require diagnosis or medical attention.

Hodder & Stoughton policy is to use papers that are natural,
renewable and recyclable products and made from wood grown in
sustainable forests. The logging and manufacturing processes are
expected to conform to the environmental regulations of the country
of origin.

Hodder & Stoughton Ltd
Carmelite House
50 Victoria Embankment
London
EC4Y 0DZ

www.hodder.co.uk

Contents

Introduction

As experts in nutritional medicine, and authors of the award-winning exposé *The Health Delusion*, we think we're well placed to sort the wheat from the chaff in matters concerning health. So when it comes to dieting, we're both serious sceptics. A bit like the seasons, or the latest fashion, fad diets come and go. While they often deliver weight loss in the short term, dieting has a spectacular failure rate in the long run. People just can't keep the weight off and they end up back where they started, more often than not with added interest. Of the hundreds of millions of people who will follow popularised diets this year less than 1 per cent will achieve permanent weight loss[1]. So disillusioned are we with their empty promises that despite the population becoming fatter, the number of people following diets is more than a third less than it was 20 years ago. Clearly something is wrong.

It would be fair to say, dieting has never been our thing. That is, until we discovered Sirtfoods, a radical new and easy way of eating which will cause you to lose weight *and* keep it off, with the added bonus of making you much healthier in the process.

What are Sirtfoods?

Over the past few years the dieting community has developed a voracious appetite for fasting diets, and with good reason. Studies show that by fasting – whether through moderate calorie restriction every day or the more severe but less frequent intermittent fasting – followers can expect to lose about 13–14lb (6kg) in 6 months and experience substantial reductions in their risk of developing disease[2].

When we fast the reduction in our body's energy stores activates what is known as the 'skinny gene' and with this a raft of positive changes ensue. Fat storage is switched off and our body stops its normal growth processes and goes into 'survival' mode. Fat burning is stimulated and the housekeeping genes involved in the repair and rejuvenation of our cells are turned on. The upshot is weight loss and improved resistance to disease.

But there is a cost attached to all of this. The reduction in energy intake provokes hunger, irritability, fatigue and loss of muscle. And that really is the elephant in the room with fasting diets; when done right, they work, but they leave many of us feeling miserable and we just don't stick to them. This leads us to the big question: is it possible to achieve this range of benefits without actually needing to undergo intense calorie restriction and its numerous drawbacks?

Enter Sirtfoods, a newly discovered group of foods. Sirtfoods are particularly rich in special nutrients that, when we consume them, are able to activate the same skinny genes in our bodies as fasting does. These genes are known as sirtuins. They first came to light in a landmark study in 2003 when researchers discovered that resveratrol, a compound found in red grape skin and red wine, dramatically increased the life span of yeast. This was the same outcome as in calorie restriction, but now no reduction in energy intake was needed[3]. Since then researchers have found that other compounds in red wine exert a similar effect, which is now believed to explain the health benefits of red wine consumption and potentially why people who drink red wine gain less weight[4].

This sparked huge interest in what other foods contain exceptionally high levels of these special nutrients capable of triggering such a profoundly beneficial effect in the body, and bit by bit, research has uncovered a collection of these powerful foods. While some of them might not be so well known to us, such as the traditional British herb lovage, which has fallen off our culinary radar, the vast majority are well known, and indeed, much enjoyed foods, such as extra virgin olive oil, red onions, parsley, chilli, kale, strawberries, walnuts, capers, tofu, cocoa, green tea, and even coffee.

Master regulators of metabolism

Since that 2003 finding excitement over the benefits of Sirtfoods has reached fever pitch. Research now shows their benefits extend further than simply mimicking the effects of caloric restriction. Sirtfoods act as master regulators of our whole metabolism, most notably having effects on fat burning while simultaneously increasing muscle and enhancing cellular fitness. The world of health research was on the cusp of the most important nutritional discovery of all time. Sadly, it took a wrong turn as the pharmaceutical industry invested hundreds of millions of pounds in researching how to turn Sirtfoods into a marketable Shangri-La pill, and the spotlight on diet was lost. We think there is something inherently wrong with that pharmaceutical approach, which tries (and so far fails) to reduce the benefits of these complex plant nutrients into a single isolated drug. Instead of waiting for the pharmaceutical industry to turn the nutrients in the food we eat into some type of alleged wonder drug (which may well never be successful anyway), we think it makes infinitely more sense to eat diets sufficiently rich in these nutrients in their natural food form to reap these exciting benefits. This became the basis for our pilot trial, as we set out to create a diet containing the richest-known sources of Sirtfoods and to observe its effects.

A common link in the world's healthiest diets

As we researched further, we discovered the best sources of Sirtfoods were found in the diets of those boasting the lowest incidence of disease and obesity rates in the world. From the Kuna American Indians, who appear immune to high blood pressure and show remarkably low rates of obesity, diabetes, cancer and early death thanks to a fantastically rich intake of the Sirtfood cocoa, to Okinawa, Japan where a buffet of Sirtfoods, svelte figures and long life all go hand in hand. In India, the voracious appetite for all things spicy, especially the Sirtfood turmeric has left cancer in its wake. And to the envy of the rest of the Western world, in a traditional Mediterranean diet, obesity simply does not prevail and chronic disease is the exception not the norm. Extra virgin olive oil, wild leafy greens, nuts, berries, red wine, dates and herbs are all potent Sirtfoods and all feature prominently in the native Mediterranean diet. The scientific world has been left in awe in light of the most recent consensus that following a Mediterranean diet is more effective than counting calories for weight loss, and more effective than pharmaceutical drugs for stopping disease[5].

Though Sirtfoods are not a mainstay of the British diet today this was not always the case. Sirtfoods used to be a staple in British kitchens, and while many have fallen off the menu, and some have vanished altogether, we will soon show that this can easily be rectified.

A modern idea in an ancient trial

Sirtfoods may be a recent nutritional discovery in the world of science but it is clear that different cultures have been experiencing their benefits throughout history. In fact it now appears that records of the benefits of Sirtfoods go way back to being the subject of the very first clinical trial ever recorded. Documented over 2,200 years ago we find it in the Book of Daniel in the Bible. What was perceived to be the best available food of the day was prescribed to keep the young men healthy and fit so they could later enter the king's service. Yet, seemingly when challenged by Daniel, a diet of only plants produced a superior outcome in just a matter of days: 'Daniel made up his mind not to let himself become ritually unclean by eating the rich food and drinking the wine of the royal court . . . So Daniel went to the guard . . . Test us for ten days, he said. Give us vegetables [plants] to eat and water to drink. Then compare us with the young men who are eating the food of the royal court, and base your decision on how we look. He agreed to let them try it for ten days. When the time was up, it was seen that they were better in appearance and fatter in flesh [muscular] than all those who had been eating the royal food. So from then on the guard let them continue to eat vegetables instead of what the king provided.'

What's really intriguing to us is the observation that along with the other benefits the plant diet increased muscle mass, an effect that would never be expected from a diet of just plants. Unless that is, those plants happen to be extremely rich Sirtfood sources. With records showing that the common plants consumed back then were similar to the Sirtfood-rich traditional Mediterranean diet, it leaves us wondering whether the Daniel trial is the stuff of fable or have we unwittingly had the answer to achieving the body and health we've always desired for over two millennia? As you are about to discover, the similarities in approach and outcome between what Daniel trialled a couple of thousand years ago and our modern-day Sirtfood Diet trial are striking.

The Sirtfood pilot study

The more we discovered about Sirtfoods, the more intrigued we became. We began to ask the question: what would happen if we gathered together this powerful set of foods and constructed a special Sirtfood Diet? In theory, we thought this would have a profound effect on weight loss and health but we knew it was mere speculation – we would have to test our ideas in the real world and generate evidence.

The chance to design and test the Sirtfood Diet came in an unlikely place. Nestled in the heart of Chelsea, London, is KX, one of Europe's most sought-after health and fitness centres. What makes KX the perfect place to trial the effects of the Sirtfood Diet is that it has its own restaurant, which gave us the opportunity not just to design the diet, but to bring it to life and test it on the fitness centre's members, with the help of KX's renowned head chef, Alessandro Verdenelli.

Our remit was clear. For seven days in a row, KX members would follow our carefully constructed Sirtfood Diet and we would meticulously track their progress from beginning to end, not just measuring their weight, but also monitoring changes in their body composition, which basically means checking how the diet affected the levels of fat and muscle in the body. Later, we added metabolic measures too, to see the effects of the diet on levels of sugar (glucose) and fats (like triglycerides and cholesterol) in the blood.

The first three days were the most intense, with food intake restricted to 1,000 calories per day. In effect, this is like a mild fast, which is important because the lower energy intake turns down growth signals in the body. Instead it encourages the body to start clearing old debris out of cells (a process known as autophagy) and kick-start fat burning. But unlike popular fasting diets, this fast was mild and gentle and much more sustainable as noted by the study's overall exceptionally high 97.5 per cent adherence rate.

Our real goal was to make a big difference to the fat-burning effects of this mild calorie restriction by packing the diet full of Sirtfoods. This was achieved by basing the daily diet on three Sirtfood-rich green juices and one Sirtfood-rich meal. We emphasised green juices because they allowed us to load up therapeutic levels of Sirtfoods, while remaining within the 1,000 calorie limit. The juices were consumed early morning, afternoon and evening, and the meal could be taken any time up until 7pm.

For the final four days of our programme at KX, calories were increased to 1,500 per day. Effectively this was only a very mild calorie deficit, but enough to keep growth signals turned down and fat-burning signals turned up. Importantly, that 1,500 calorie diet was jam-packed full of Sirtfoods, consisting of two Sirtfood-rich juices and two Sirtfood-rich meals per day.

The remarkable results

The Sirtfood Diet was trialled by 40 and completed by 39 members at KX. Of these 39, two in the trial were obese, 15 were overweight and 22 had a normal/healthy BMI. The study had a fairly even gender split, with 21 women and 18 men. Being members of a health club they were more likely to exercise and be aware of healthy eating than the general population, before they started.

A trick of many diets is to use a heavily overweight and unhealthy sample of people to show their benefits, as at first they lose weight the quickest and most dramatically, essentially fluffing up their results. Our logic was the opposite: if we obtained good results with this relatively healthy group, it would set the minimum benchmark of what was achievable.

The results far exceeded our already high expectations. Results were consistent and astounding: an average 7lb (3.2kg) of weight loss in seven days after accounting for muscle gain. No participant failed to see improvements in body composition. All of this was achieved without severe calorie restriction or gruelling exercise regimes.

Here's what we found:

- participants achieved dramatic and rapid results, losing an average of 7lb (3.2kg) in seven days
- rather than lose muscle, muscle mass was either maintained or increased
- participants rarely felt hungry
- participants felt an increased sense of vitality and well-being
- participants reported looking better and healthier

CASE STUDY

Jadis, a 32-year-old marketing executive from London, was worried about her waistline and wanted to be in the best possible shape for her impending wedding day. 'I have diabetes in my family, so I've always been aware of the need to stay trim. But even though I eat well and work out regularly, I just couldn't shift those few extra pounds around my middle – precisely the area my dress was going to highlight.'

After seven days of following our Sirtfood trial, the results, she says, were 'amazing'. Jadis had lost over 6lb (2.7kg), which included putting on nearly 2lb (900g) of muscle, despite engaging in virtually no exercise in that time. She reported never feeling hungry, increased energy and to top it off she showed improvements in her diabetes risk factors of sugar and fats in the blood. A check-in with Jadis a week later, just before her wedding, showed her results continued to improve with a further 2lb 6oz (1.1kg) weight loss.

What's so good about muscle-adjusted weight loss?

Losing 7lb (3.2kg) in seven days is good by anyone's standard, but what made our Sirtfood Diet trial so different was the type of weight loss and changes in body composition we were seeing.

Typically when people lose weight they will lose some fat but they will also lose muscle – this is what occurs on practically every other diet that has gone before. So if someone loses 7lb (3.2kg) on the scales in a week through normal 'dieting', you can be pretty confident that at least 2lb (900g) of it is muscle. And so that's exactly what we expected when we came to measure our participants' body composition too. Much to our surprise, as the body composition results trickled through, we began to see a startling finding. While it was common to see weight loss of 7lb (3.2kg) on the scales, something else was occurring a lot more often. For 64 per cent of our study participants, the losses on the scales initially appeared more disappointing than this, albeit still very impressive, with a weight loss of just over 5lb (2.3kg). But when body composition tests were performed we were gobsmacked. Muscle mass was not just maintained in these participants, it had increased. The average muscle gain for this group was almost 2lb (900g), giving what is called a 'muscle gain adjusted weight loss' of 7lb (3.2kg). As we are about to discover, this is an infinitely more favourable type of weight loss than losing fat and muscle together.

This was a remarkable finding, especially given that the combination of mild calorie restriction and no increase in exercise would, under normal circumstances, be disastrous for maintaining muscle. There had to be another explanation for this astonishing outcome: the powerful metabolic effects of Sirtfoods. Not only are Sirtfoods able to activate fat burning, but they also promote muscle growth, maintenance and repair. In effect, our diet rich in Sirtfoods allowed participants to lose fat, without the collateral damage of losing muscle.

You may be asking yourself why this is so important. Firstly, it means you'll look much better. Stripping away the fat, but retaining muscle, leads to a more desirable toned and athletic physique. And even more importantly, you'll stay looking good. Skeletal muscle is the major factor that accounts for our body's daily energy expenditure. This means the more muscle you have, the more energy you burn, even when resting. With typical dieting, weight loss is made up of fat loss and muscle loss, and with that we see a marked decline in the metabolic rate. This primes the body for weight regain when more normal eating habits are resumed. But by keeping hold of your muscle mass with Sirtfoods, you burn more fat with a minimal drop in metabolic rate. This provides the perfect foundation for long-term weight-loss success.

Additionally, muscle mass and function is a predictor of well-being, and maintaining muscle prevents the development of chronic diseases, such as diabetes and osteoporosis, as well as keeping us mobile into older age. Importantly, it also appears to keep us happier, with scientists suggesting that the way sirtuins maintain muscle even has benefits for stress-related disorders, including reducing depression[6].

With previous diets comes the controversial axiom that you cannot be slim and have enhanced longevity without a loss of muscle. To us this just makes no sense. Muscle mass and function is a key indicator of health and well-being and should be consistent with looking great and being healthy. The Sirtfood Diet lays this contention firmly to rest.

Britain's glamourites and sports stars come flocking

Any diet that can so powerfully promote fat loss and improve body composition has many useful applications. While the diet was still a well-kept secret confined to a chic gym in the heart of one of London's most exclusive postcodes, word about our work was spreading, and Britain's glamourites and sports stars wanted in. We began applying the principles of the Sirtfood Diet to sporting stars, from boxers to rugby players to sailors, all of whom represented Britain at the highest level, from Olympic heroes, right up to those who had received knighthoods in recognition of their sporting success. Not only did these athletes see body composition results that they had never before achieved in their careers, but the improved performance opened up new opportunities for sporting success.

One such example is the iconic British heavyweight boxing champion David Haye. A stream of injuries left David in the boxing doldrums and many wondering if he would ever box again. When we first met him, he was carrying over 22lb (10kg) in excess body fat. Getting David back into shape and into the ring initially looked like an impossible feat, but David is back and setting himself for another world title challenge with a body composition and functionality he has never achieved before. In David's own words, 'Sirtfoods have been a revelation to my diet. Introducing Sirtfoods has allowed me to attain a body composition and well-being previously unimaginable, paving the way for my return to the ring and regaining my title as heavyweight champion of the world.'

How the Sirtfood Diet will work for you

The good news is, you don't need to be an elite athlete, or even remotely sporty, to reap these benefits. We've taken everything we've learnt about Sirtfoods, both through the pilot study at KX and through our work with elite athletes, and adapted it to create the Sirtfood Diet, a diet that will work for anyone who wants to lose weight and become healthier.

It doesn't require you to perform severe calorie restriction, nor does it demand gruelling exercise regimes (although of course, staying generally active is a good thing). It is neither expensive nor time-consuming, and all the foods we recommend are widely available. The only piece of kit you'll need is a juicer. Plus, unlike every other diet out there that focuses on what you should be excluding, the Sirtfood Diet focuses on what you should be including.

CASE STUDY

One advocate of the Sirtfood Diet approach is the former top model and now TV celebrity chef and food writer Lorraine Pascale. As she explains, the beauty of Sirtfoods is in their simplicity and convenience: 'This plan is easy to follow. We all know that eating healthily can be quite expensive, so is often off-putting to some people. I believe in trying to eat more of the good stuff to try and crowd out the naughtier stuff. The great thing about Sirtfoods is that lots of them are foods we eat every day anyway. Most Sirtfoods are very accessible and can be easily added to family food for everyone's enjoyment.'

OVERVIEW OF PHASE 1

Phase 1 of the Sirtfood Diet is the hyper-success phase. Over seven days you'll follow our clinically proven method for losing 7lb (3.2kg). We'll give you a step-by-step guide, including a menu plan and recipes.

During the first three days, your calorie intake will be restricted to a maximum of 1,000 calories per day. This will consist of three Sirtfood-rich green juices, plus one full meal rich in Sirtfoods per day.

For days four to seven, your calorie intake will increase to a maximum of 1,500 calories. Each day will comprise two Sirtfood-rich green juices and two Sirtfood-rich meals. By the end of the seven days, you can expect to have lost an average of 7lb (3.2kg).

Despite the reduction in calories participants do not feel unduly hungry, with the calorie limit representing a guideline rather than a target. Even in the most intensive phase calorie restriction is not severe compared to most fasting recommendations. With Sirtfoods having natural satiating effects most people actually find themselves being pleasantly satisfied and full.

OVERVIEW OF PHASE 2

Phase 2 is the 14-day maintenance phase, where despite not focusing on cutting calories, you will consolidate your weight-loss results and continue to lose weight steadily. The key to success in this phase is to keep eating a wealth of Sirtfoods which is made easy with our 14-day sample diet plan and accompanying recipes. This phase will see you eating three balanced Sirtfood-rich meals each day, along with a 'maintenance' Sirtfood green juice.

A plan for life

The beauty of the Sirtfood Diet is that you don't have to be constantly dieting. Phase 1 and Phase 2 can be repeated periodically for a fat-loss boost, if needed. For some that might be every three months, for others it might be once a year. That just leaves you to get on with the rest of your life, slimmer and healthier than before, while continuing to enjoy the bounty of health benefits that a diet rich in Sirtfoods brings. In fact, such is the universal application of Sirtfoods that they can be comfortably incorporated into any existing dietary regimen that you follow, whether that be vegan, gluten-free, low-carb, paleo, intermittent fasting and so on (for more on this see chapter 11). Incorporating significant amounts of Sirtfoods will amplify the weight loss and health benefits of all of those approaches.

For us, the real key to success is achieving results that last a lifetime, and this is where the Sirtfood Diet really shines. Equipped with your new-found knowledge of Sirtfoods, we will show you how to take your normal day-to-day diet, and through some smart food swaps and tweaks, turn it into a sustainable Sirtfood-rich way of eating that you can follow long term. By understanding the basic tenets of a healthy diet and supplementation, with practical tips for integrating more Sirtfoods into your everyday diet, you will be set to reap the positive benefits for the rest of your life.

Here's what the Sirtfood Diet will do for you:

- drive weight loss from fat, not muscle
- prime your body for long-term weight-loss success
- ensure you look and feel better and have more energy
- prevent you having to endure severe fasting or extreme hunger
- free you of gruelling exercise regimes
- be a springboard for a longer, healthier, disease-free life

SUMMARY

- Sirtfoods contain a newly discovered group of nutrients, found in plants, which provide the benefits of fasting without its shortcomings. Examples of Sirtfoods include extra virgin olive oil, capers, red onions, parsley, kale, walnuts, strawberries, chilli, soy products, cocoa, green tea and coffee.

- Sirtfoods go beyond the effects of fasting, acting as master regulators of metabolism, not only stimulating fat burning but promoting muscle gain and increases in cellular fitness.

- Sirtfoods have been found to be key ingredients in traditional diets associated with markedly less obesity and disease and increased longevity, such as the Mediterranean and Japanese diets.

- By combining a diet packed with Sirtfoods with moderate calorie restriction, the Sirtfood Diet has been clinically proven to achieve a weight loss of 7lb (3.2kg) in seven days. This includes maintaining or increasing muscle, as well as programming the body for lasting and sustainable weight-loss success.

- Participants of the Sirtfood Diet report feeling and looking better as well as having more energy.

- Sirtfoods have become the successful diet strategy for a number of elite athletes, enabling them to reach their body composition and fitness goals.

- The Sirtfood Diet is a diet of inclusion that celebrates just how powerful correct nutrition can be. Over the course of the next few chapters we will lay out exactly how you too can reap the amazing benefits from eating Sirtfoods.

The Science of Sirtuins

What makes the Sirtfood Diet so powerful is its ability to switch on an ancient family of genes that exists in each of us. The name for this family of genes is sirtuin. Sirtuins are special because they orchestrate processes deep within our cells that influence such important things as our ability to burn fat, our susceptibility – or not – to disease, and ultimately even our lifespan. So profound is the effect of sirtuins that they are now referred to as 'master metabolic regulators'[7]. In essence, exactly what anyone wanting to shed some pounds and live a long and healthy life would want to be in charge of.

Of mice and men

Understandably, sirtuins have become the subject of intense scientific research in recent years. The first sirtuin was discovered back in 1984 in yeast, and interest really took off over the course of the next three decades when it was revealed that sirtuin activation increases lifespan, first in yeast, and then all the way up to mice[8].

Why the excitement? Because from yeast to humans and everything in between, the fundamental principles of cellular metabolism are nearly identical. If you can manipulate something as tiny as a budding yeast and see a benefit, then repeat it in higher organisms such as mice, the potential exists for the same benefits to be realised in humans.

An appetite for fasting?

Which brings us nicely on to fasting. The lifelong restriction of food intake has been consistently shown to extend the life expectancy of lower organisms and mammals[9]. A remarkable finding, which is the basis for the practice of caloric restriction among some people, where daily calorie intake is reduced by about 20–30 per cent; as well as its popularised off-shoot, intermittent fasting, which has become a successful weight-loss diet, made famous by the likes of the 5:2 Diet. While we still await proof of increased lifespan for humans from these practices, there is proof of benefits for what we might term 'healthspan' – chronic diseases drop and fat starts to melt away[10].

But let's be honest, no matter how big the benefits, fasting week in, week out, is a gruelling business that most of us aren't willing to sign up to. Even if we do, most of us can't stick to it. On top of this there are drawbacks to fasting, especially when we follow it long term. In the introduction we mentioned the side effects of hunger, irritability, fatigue and muscle loss. But in addition, ongoing fasting regimes could put us at risk of malnutrition, affecting our well-being due to a lowered intake of essential nutrients. Fasting regimes are also wholly unsuitable for large proportions of the population such as children, in pregnancy, and very possibly the elderly. While there are clearly established benefits to fasting, it's not the magic bullet we would like it to be. It had us asking, is this really the way nature intended for us to be thin *and* healthy? Surely there's a better way . . .

Our breakthrough came when we discovered that the profound benefits from caloric restriction and fasting were mediated through activation of our ancient sirtuin genes[11]. To better understand this, it might be helpful to think about sirtuins as the guardians at the crossroads between energy status and longevity. What they do there is respond to stresses.

When energy is in short supply, exactly as we see in caloric restriction, there is an increase in stress on our cells. This is sensed by the sirtuins, which then get switched on and broadcast a constellation of powerful signals that radically alter the way cells behave. Sirtuins ramp up our metabolism, increase the efficiency of our muscles, switch on fat burning, reduce inflammation and repair any damage in our cells. In effect, sirtuins make us fitter, leaner and healthier.

> In humans, there are seven different sirtuins (Sirt-1 to Sirt-7). Of these, Sirt-1 and Sirt-3 are the two most important sirtuins involved in energy balance. While Sirt-1 is found throughout the body, Sirt-3 is predominantly found in our mitochondria – the energy powerhouses of our cells. Together their activation gives us the many benefits we are looking to achieve.

A zeal for exercise?

It's not just caloric restriction and fasting that activate sirtuins; exercise does too[12]. Just like in fasting, sirtuins orchestrate the profound benefits of exercise. But while we are encouraged to engage in regular moderate exercise for its multitude of benefits, it is not the means through which we are meant to focus our weight-loss efforts. Research shows that our body has evolved ways to naturally adjust and reduce the amount of energy we expend when we exercise[13], meaning that in order for exercise to be an effective weight-loss intervention we need to commit substantial time and strenuous effort. That gruelling exercise regimes are the way nature intended us to maintain a healthy weight is even more dubious in the light of research now suggesting that too much exercise can be harmful – weakening our immune systems, damaging the heart and contributing to an early death[14, 15].

ENTER SIRTFOODS

So far we have discovered that if we want to lose weight and be healthy, the key is to activate our sirtuin genes. Up until now the two known ways to achieve this have been fasting and exercise. Alas, the amounts needed for successful weight loss come with their drawbacks, and for most of us are simply incompatible with how we live life in the twenty-first century. Fortunately, there is a newly discovered, groundbreaking means of activating our sirtuin genes in the best possible way: Sirtfoods. As we will soon learn lots more about, these are the wonder foods particularly rich in specific natural plant chemicals which have the power to speak to our sirtuin genes, switching them on. In essence they mimic the effects of fasting and exercise and in doing so bring remarkable benefits for burning fat, building muscle and boosting health, which were previously unattainable.

SUMMARY

- Each of us possesses an ancient family of genes called sirtuins.

- Sirtuins are master metabolic regulators that control our ability to burn fat and stay healthy.

- Sirtuins act as energy sensors within our cells, and get activated when a shortage of energy is detected.

- Fasting and exercise both activate our sirtuin genes, but can be hard to stick to and even have drawbacks.

- There is a new groundbreaking way to activate our sirtuin genes: Sirtfoods.

- By eating a diet rich in Sirtfoods you can mimic the effects of fasting and exercise, and achieve the body you want.

2

Fighting Fat

One of the dramatic findings from our pilot study of the Sirtfood Diet was not just the amount of weight the participants lost, which was impressive enough – it was the *type* of weight loss that really got us excited. What really grabbed our attention was the fact that many people were losing weight without losing any muscle. In fact, it was not uncommon to see people gain muscle. This left us with an inescapable conclusion: fat was just melting away.

Normally, achieving significant fat loss requires a considerable sacrifice, either severely cutting back on calories, engaging in super-human levels of exercise, or both. But contrary to that, our participants either maintained or reduced their exercise levels, and didn't even report feeling particularly hungry. In fact, some even struggled to eat all the food that was provided for them.

How is this even possible? It's only when we understand what happens to our fat cells when sirtuin activity is increased that we can begin to make sense of these remarkable findings.

Lean genes

Mice that have been genetically engineered to have high levels of Sirt-1, the sirtuin gene that drives fat loss, are leaner and more metabolically active[16], whereas mice lacking Sirt-1 are fatter and have more metabolic disease[17]. When we look at humans, levels of Sirt-1 have been found to be markedly lower in the body fat of obese people than their healthy-weight counterparts[18, 19]. In contrast, people with increased Sirt-1 gene activity are leaner and more resistant to weight gain[20].

Stack all that up and you start to get a sense of just how important sirtuins are for determining whether we stay lean or get fat, and why by increasing sirtuin activity you can achieve such amazing results. This is because through sirtuins we get benefits on multiple levels, starting at the very root of it all; the genes that control weight gain.

To better understand this we need to delve deeper into what happens in our cells that causes us to gain weight.

CASE STUDY

Kate is a housewife and mother to two young children in her mid-thirties. With a body fat of over 25 per cent she was classed as 'acceptable' but was unhappy as she was still carrying those extra few pregnancy pounds around the middle. Despite being quite active – exercising in the gym when she could and being constantly on her feet with two energy-filled children to look after – her weight did not shift. Diet-wise she had always tried to eat quite healthily, and if anything stated that she ate too little instead of too much, with it not being uncommon for her to skip a meal to ensure the children were looked after.

The ease and convenience of the Sirtfood Diet made it perfect for her to try it out, and she achieved fantastic results. By the end of the week Kate was down 6lb 8oz (3kg) on the scales and had gained 1lb (450g) in muscle. Her body fat was now 22 per cent, putting her in the 'fit' range that she so desired.

Fat busting

We're going to explain this in terms of a Hollywood drug-ring film. The flooding of the streets with drugs is the flooding of our body with fat. The drug pushers on the street corners are the equivalent of the reactions in our body that peddle weight gain. But in reality, they are only the low-level thugs. Behind it all is the true villain masterminding the whole operation, directing every deal the peddlers make. In our film, this villain is called PPAR-γ (peroxisome proliferator-activated receptor-γ). PPAR-γ orchestrates the fat-gain process by switching on the genes that are needed to start synthesising and storing fat[21]. To stop the proliferation of fat you must cut the supply. Stop PPAR-γ, and you effectively stop fat gain.

Enter our hero, Sirt-1, who rises up to bring down the villain. With the villain securely locked up, there is no one to pull the strings and the whole fat-gain organisation crumbles. With the activity of PPAR-γ halted, Sirt-1 moves its attentions to 'cleaning the streets'. Not only is this done by shutting down the production and storage of fat as we've seen, but it actually changes our metabolism so we start ridding our body of excess fat[22]. Just like every good crime-fighting hero, Sirt-1 has a sidekick, a key regulator in our cells known as PGC-1α. This powerfully stimulates the creation of what are known as mitochondria. These are the tiny energy factories that exist within each of our cells – they power the body. The more mitochondria we have, the more energy we can produce. But not only does PGC-1α promote more mitochondria, it also encourages them to burn fat as the fuel of choice to make the energy. So, on the one hand fat storage is blocked, on the other, fat burning is increased.

CASE STUDY

Kathleen Baird-Murray, a beauty columnist for the *Financial Times*, and a writer for *Vogue* and *Porter* magazines, is no stranger to the latest en vogue diets. With her holidays coming up, she followed and reported on the latest diet trends for her column, including the Sirtfood Diet. Time-constrained, she followed it for six instead of seven days. And she still managed a fantastic 6lb 13oz (3.1kg) weight loss, taking her from 'overweight' to 'normal weight'. She was 'so impressed' with the diet, saying that she enjoyed eating healthy food that was filling, but also delicious, and appreciated the renewed energy she felt.

WAT or BAT?

So far we've looked at the effects of Sirt-1 on fat loss on a well-known type of fat called white adipose tissue (WAT).

This is the type of fat associated with weight gain. It specialises in storage and expansion, is horribly stubborn and secretes a host of inflammatory chemicals that resist fat burning and encourage further fat accumulation, making us overweight and obese. This is why weight gain often starts slowly but can snowball so quickly.

But there is another intriguing angle to the sirtuin story, involving a lesser-known type of fat, known as brown adipose tissue (BAT), which behaves very differently. In complete contrast to white adipose tissue, BAT is beneficial to us and wants to get used up. Brown adipose tissue actually helps us expend energy and has evolved in mammals to allow them to dissipate large amounts of energy in the form of heat. This is known as a thermogenic effect and is critical to small mammals to help them survive in cold temperatures. In humans, babies also possess significant amounts of brown adipose tissue, although it reduces soon after birth, leaving smaller amounts in adults.

Here is where Sirt-1 activation does something truly amazing. It switches on genes in our white adipose tissue so that it morphs and takes on the properties of brown adipose tissue in what is called a 'browning effect'[23]. That means our fat stores start to behave in an altogether different way – instead of storing energy they start to mobilise it for disposal.

As we can see, sirtuin activation has potent direct action on fat cells, encouraging fat to melt away. But it doesn't end there. Sirtuins also positively influence the most relevant hormones involved in weight control. Sirtuin activation improves insulin activity[24]. This helps to reduce insulin resistance – the inability of our cells to respond properly to insulin – which is heavily implicated in weight gain. Sirt-1 also enhances the release and activity of our thyroid hormones[25], which share many overlapping roles in boosting our metabolism and ultimately the rate at which we burn fat.

CASE STUDY

James is a busy entrepreneur in his late thirties. His hectic schedule had left him feeling run-down and exhausted and his weight had gradually crept up and now exceeded 14½ stone (92kg), putting him in the obese category. With a family history of diabetes, James wanted to do something to ensure that wasn't his future fate. But despite fitting in exercise around his work commitments as best he could, his weight was inexorably creeping up.

After seven days of the Sirtfood Diet James had lost 7lb 4oz (3.3kg). While still classified as obese, this was the springboard James needed to make longer-term changes. It made him realise that weight gain wasn't inevitable and he could do something about it. Better news was to come in the form of a very substantial reduction in his fasting blood sugar level, which had been approaching pre-diabetic levels.

Appetite control

There was one thing we couldn't wrap our heads around in our pilot study: despite a significant reduction in calories participants didn't really get hungry. In fact some individuals struggled to eat all the food provided.

One of the big advantages of the Sirtfood Diet is that we can achieve great benefits without the need for long-term, intense fasting. The very first week of the diet is the hyper-success phase, where we combine moderate fasting with an abundance of powerful Sirtfoods for a double blow to fat. And like all fasting regimens we expected some reports of hunger here. But we got absolutely none!

As we trawled through research we found the answer. In contrast to what happens elsewhere in the body, when we fast, Sirt-1 activity in a part of the brain called the hypothalamus decreases[26]. The result of this is an increase in appetite and reduction in the amount of energy we expend. This makes perfect sense, as it is something most of us will have experienced. Go a period without eating and hunger kicks in and energy levels wane. But by combining fasting with our sirtuin-activating diet, it seems we maintained the Sirt-1 activity in the hypothalamus, cancelling out the negative effect of fasting, and preventing hunger from kicking in. It would also explain why our participants, many of whom have mentally demanding jobs and physically demanding lifestyles didn't report drops in energy levels. Many actually reported increased energy.

Interestingly, scientists have shown that reductions in Sirt-1 in the hypothalamus also occur in old age, and from consumption of a high-fat–high-sugar diet[27]. This explains why we find it easier to gain fat and become less energetic in later life, and why despite being full of energy in the form of calories, we eat more yet feel lethargic when consuming high-fat–high-sugar foods.

As we will see later, Sirtfoods also have powerful effects on our taste centres, meaning we get much more pleasure and satisfaction from our food and do not therefore fall into the trap of over-eating to feel satisfied.

Even for the most dedicated dieters, sirtuins are likely to be a brand-new concept. Yet, as master regulators of our metabolism, targeting sirtuins is the cornerstone of any successful weight-loss diet. Tragically, the very nature of our modern society, with abundant food and sedentary lifestyles, creates a perfect storm for switching off our sirtuin activity, and we see the fallout of this all around us.

The good news is that now we know what sirtuins are,

how they control fat storage and promote fat burning, and most importantly how to switch them on. And with this revolutionary breakthrough, finally the answer to effective and sustained weight loss is yours for the taking.

CASE STUDY

Anthony Ogogo is a British Olympic medal winner and professional middleweight boxer. After a year out recovering from surgery he was keen to get his return spot on, including his nutrition.

Anthony says: 'When I first met Aidan and Glen, I was 12st 13lb (82kg) and needing to make the 11st 6lb (72.5kg) limit to fight as a professional middleweight. This had always been a struggle in the past. A lot of boxers use temporary measures to lose weight, but they don't last long term and you don't feel good doing them. I didn't want that. I wanted sustained and effective weight loss, one that targeted fat over muscle, kept me sharp, strong and full of energy. Through introducing Sirtfoods I very quickly achieved this weight loss and felt better entering the ring than I ever had done before.'

SUMMARY

- Fat melts away on the Sirtfood Diet. This is because sirtuins have the power to determine whether we stay lean or get fat.

- Activating Sirt-1 inhibits PPAR-γ, blocking the production and storage of fat.

- Activating Sirt-1 also turns on PGC-1α, which makes more energy factories in our cells and increases fat burning.

- Activating Sirt-1 even gets our fat cells that specialise in energy storage to behave differently and start disposing of energy.

- You are unlikely to feel hungry on the Sirtfood Diet because it helps to regulate appetite in the brain.

3

Masters of Muscle

One of the findings from our pilot trial that really got us intrigued was that the muscle mass of the participants didn't drop; in fact it often increased. The average increase in muscle for the study was just over 1lb (450g), with many participants seeing a gain in the region of 2lb (900g). This was completely unexpected. The classic trade-off for any diet that limits calories is that you can kiss goodbye to some muscle as well as fat. This is not surprising when you consider that when we deprive the body of energy, cells shift from 'growth' mode to 'survival' mode and will use the protein from muscle for fuel.

Sirtuins and muscle mass

There is a family of genes in the body which act as guardians of our muscle and halt its breakdown when under stress; the sirtuins[28]. Sirt-1 is a potent inhibitor of muscle breakdown. As long as Sirt-1 is activated, even when we are fasting, muscle breakdown is prevented and we continue to burn fat for fuel.

But the benefits of Sirt-1 don't end with preserving muscle mass. Sirtuins actually work to increase our skeletal muscle mass[29-31]. To explain how this phenomenon works we need to venture into the exciting world of stem cells. Our muscle contains a special type of stem cell, called satellite cells, which control its growth and regeneration. Satellite cells just sit there quietly most of the time, but they are activated when muscle gets damaged or stressed. This is how our muscles get bigger through activities like weight training. Sirt-1 is essential for activating satellite cells and without its activity muscles are significantly smaller as they no longer have the capacity to develop or regenerate properly[32]. However, by increasing Sirt-1 activity, we give a boost to our satellite cells, which encourages muscle growth and recovery.

Sirtfoods versus fasting

This leads us to a big question: if sirtuin activation increases muscle mass, then why do we lose muscle when we fast? After all, fasting activates our sirtuin genes as well. And herein lies one of the massive drawbacks of fasting.

Bear with us, while we delve into how this works. Not all skeletal muscle is created equal. We have two main types, conveniently called type-1 and type-2. Type-1 muscle is used for longer duration activities, whereas type-2 muscle is used for short bursts of more intense activity. And here's where it gets intriguing, fasting *only* increases Sirt-1 activity in type-1 muscle fibres, not type-2[33]. So type-1 muscle fibre size is maintained and even noticeably increases when we fast[34]. Sadly, in complete contrast to what happens in type-1 fibres during fasting, Sirt-1 rapidly declines in type-2 fibres. This means fat burning slows down, and instead muscle starts to break down to provide fuel.

So fasting is a double-edged sword for muscles, with our type-2 fibres taking a hit. Type-2 fibres are what comprise the bulk of our muscle definition. So even though our type-1 fibre mass increases we still see an overall significant loss of muscle with fasting. If we could stop their break-down it would not only make us look good aesthetically but also help promote further fat loss. And the way to do this is to combat the drop in Sirt-1 in type-2 muscle fibre brought about by fasting.

In an elegant mice study, researchers at Harvard Medical School put this to the test, and showed that by stimulating Sirt-1 activity in type-2 fibres while fasting, the signals for muscle breakdown were switched off and muscle loss didn't occur[35].

The researchers then went one step further and tested

the effects of increased Sirt-1 activity on muscle when the mice were fed rather than fasted, and discovered that it triggered very rapid muscle growth. Within just a week, muscle fibres with increased levels of Sirt-1 activity showed an astounding 20 per cent increase in weight[36].

While much milder in effect, these findings are very similar to the outcome of our Sirtfood Diet trial. By increasing Sirt-1 activity through eating a diet rich in Sirtfoods, the majority of participants had no muscle loss, and for many, with it only being a moderate fast, muscle mass actually increased.

CASE STUDY

David 'the Hayemaker' Haye is a former world heavyweight boxing champion. After being out of the ring for three years with a career-threatening shoulder injury, he is now successfully lining up his comeback to reclaim the title of world champion.

David has earned a reputation as one of the most gifted boxers in the world but in the heavyweight category he often faced opponents that carried an additional 1½–3 stone (10–20kg) more muscle than him. Plus, having been out of action for so long with an injury meant that he was also carrying over 1½ stone (10kg) more body fat than an elite boxing champion in this category should.

What was important to him for his return to the ring was to increase muscle mass while losing fat. An avid proponent of plant-based diets he whole-heartedly adopted the Sirtfood approach, and the results quickly followed. In David's own words: 'Sirtfoods have been a revelation to my diet. Introducing Sirtfoods has allowed me to attain a body composition and well-being previously unim-aginable, paving the way for my return to the ring and regaining my title as heavyweight champion of the world. I have always endorsed the virtues of eating plants, and the discovery of Sirtfoods shows just how powerful they are and why we should eat more of them. If anyone asks me my number one tip for getting in great shape my answer is to start eating a Sirtfood-rich diet.'

Keeping muscles young

And it's not just muscle size. The prolific effects of Sirt-1 on muscle extend to how they function too. As muscle ages, its ability to activate Sirt-1 declines. This makes it less responsive to the benefits of exercise and more prone to damage from free radicals and inflammation, which results in what is known as oxidative stress. Muscles gradually wither, get weaker and fatigue more easily. But if we can increase activation of Sirt-1 we can stop the age-related decline[37–39].

Indeed by activating Sirt-1 to stop the loss of muscle mass and function we normally see with aging, we see multiple knock-on health benefits, including halting bone loss, preventing an increase in chronic systemic inflammation (known as inflammaging) as well as improving mobility and overall quality of life.

Don't be fooled into thinking these benefits only apply to the elderly, far from it. By the age of 25, the effects of aging can begin and muscle slowly erodes, with 10 per cent of muscle lost by age 40 (even though overall weight tends to increase) and a 40 per cent loss by age 70. Yet evidence is growing that this can all be prevented and reversed by stimulating our sirtuin genes.

Muscle loss, growth and function; sirtuin activity plays a pivotal role in it all. Stack it up, and it's no wonder that in a recent review in the prestigious medical journal *Nature*, sirtuins were described as master regulators of muscle growth, with increasing sirtuin activation cited as one of the promising emerging avenues for combating muscle loss, and thus increasing quality of life as well as reducing disease and deaths[40].

Viewed in the context of the powerful effects our sirtuin genes can have on muscles, the shock results of our pilot trial no longer seemed so shocking. We began to realise it was possible to fuel weight loss while feeding our muscles, all through a Sirtfood-rich diet.

But that's just the start. In the next chapter we will see the benefits of Sirtfoods extend so much further, to all aspects of health and quality of life.

SUMMARY

- Despite losing weight, we found that people following the Sirtfood Diet either maintained or even gained muscle. This is because sirtuins are master regulators of muscle.

- By activating sirtuins it is possible both to prevent muscle breakdown and promote muscle regeneration.

- Activating Sirt-1 can also help to prevent the gradual loss of muscle that we see with aging.

- Not only will activating your sirtuin genes make you look leaner, it will help you stay healthier and function better as you age.

4

Well-being Wonders

Whichever way you look at it, we're losing our battle with the bulge. Obesity rates are exploding and a host of obesity-related diseases are on the rise. Right now, more than one in three people has heart disease, with an incredible six in 10 having high blood pressure. One in 10 has diabetes, and another four are on the verge of getting it. If you see two women over the age of 50, one of them is going to have an osteoporotic fracture. Two out of every five people will be diagnosed with cancer at some stage in their lives. And in the average time it takes you to read a single page of this book, a new case of Alzheimer's will develop – and that's in the USA alone. Despite all the amazing advances in modern medicine, society is getting fatter and sicker – 70 per cent of all deaths are due to chronic disease, a truly shocking statistic. Radical change is needed, and fast.

Yet, as we have seen, we can begin to change all of this. By activating our ancient sirtuin genes we can burn fat and build a leaner and stronger body. And with sirtuins at the hub of our metabolism, master programmers of our biology, their importance extends far beyond just body composition alone, to every facet of our well-being.

Sirtuins and the 70 per cent

Think of a disease that you associate with getting old and the chances are a lack of sirtuin activity in the body is involved. For example, sirtuin activation is great for heart health, protecting the muscle cells in the heart and generally helping the heart muscle function better[41]. It also improves how our arteries work, helps us handle cholesterol more efficiently, and protects against the clogging up of our arteries known as atherosclerosis[42].

How about diabetes? Sirtuin activation increases the amount of insulin that can be secreted and helps it work more effectively in the body[43]. As it happens, one of the most popular anti-diabetic drugs, metformin, relies on Sirt-1 for its beneficial effect. Indeed, one pharmaceutical company is currently investigating adding natural sirtuin activators to metformin treatment for diabetics, with results from animal studies showing a staggering 83 per cent reduction in the dose of metformin needed for the same effects[44].

When it comes to the brain, sirtuins are involved again, with sirtuin activity found to be lower in Alzheimer's patients.

In contrast, sirtuin activation improves communication signals in the brain, enhances cognitive function and reduces brain inflammation. This stops the build-up of amyloid-β production and tau protein aggregation, two of the main damaging things we see occurring in the brains of Alzheimer's patients[45,46].

Bones are next. Osteoblasts are a special type of cell in our bones responsible for building new bone. The more osteoblasts we have, the stronger our bones. Sirtuin activation not only promotes the production of osteoblast cells, but also increases their survival[47]. This makes sirtuin activation essential for lifelong bone health.

Cancer has been a much more controversial area for sirtuin research but the latest shows that sirtuin activation helps to suppress cancer tumours[48]. While there is still more to learn on this particular topic, as we will soon see, those cultures who eat the most Sirtfoods have the lowest cancer rates.

Heart disease, diabetes, dementia, osteoporosis and very probably cancer; it's an impressive list of diseases that can be prevented by activating sirtuins. It may come as no surprise to find out that cultures already eating plenty of Sirtfoods as part of their traditional diets experience a longevity and well-being most of us could barely imagine, which you'll hear more on very soon.

That leaves us with an exciting conclusion: simply by adding the world's most potent Sirtfoods into your diet, and making that a lifelong habit, you too can experience this level of well-being – and more – all while getting the physique you want.

CASE STUDY

David Carr is a professional athlete with Land Rover BAR, the British sailing team being led by Sir Ben Ainslie to win the prestigious America's Cup for Britain for the first time ever.

David trains like a top athlete and his diet could only be regarded as healthy, including taking supplements. Yet in his own words he was 'always the fat athlete' and it irked him that he ate better and trained harder than many of the athletes around him, yet they were leaner. Despite all his exercise and good diet, he also showed risk factors for metabolic disease with high levels of blood sugar, cholesterol and other fats in his blood.

With a Sirtfood-rich diet, including a Sirtfood drink each morning, as the cornerstone of his nutritional plan, David experienced tremendous results. Within 6 months David was down from 16st 5lb (104kg) to his target weight of 14st 9lb (93kg), an incredible 24lb (11kg) weight loss. His body fat percentage had dropped by half to 7 per cent, marking him as elite. And in his own words 'every time I do something aerobic I set a personal best and I am stronger than ever'. Not only did he now look like a top athlete, something else was evident:

he also looked so much healthier. And his blood tests backed it up. Tests showed David experienced:

- a 45 per cent reduction in 'bad' LDL cholesterol
- a 29 per cent increase in 'good' HDL cholesterol
- an 80 per cent drop in triglycerides (fats in the blood)
- a decrease in blood sugar levels that took him back down to normal from the brink of prediabetes

By basing his nutritional plan around Sirtfoods, David can not only compete at his best, but has completely reversed his future risk of heart disease and diabetes.

SUMMARY

- Despite all the advances in modern medicine, as a society we're getting fatter and sicker.

- Seventy per cent of all deaths are due to chronic disease, with low sirtuin activity implicated in the vast majority.

- By activating sirtuins, you can prevent or forestall the major chronic diseases of the Western world.

- By packing your diet full of Sirtfoods you too can enjoy the same level of well-being as the healthiest and longest-living populations on the planet.

Sirtfoods

So far we have discovered that sirtuins are an ancient family of genes with the power to help us burn fat, build muscle and keep us super-healthy. It is well established that sirtuins can be switched on through caloric restriction, fasting and exercise, but there is another revolutionary way to achieve this: food. We refer to the foods most powerful at activating sirtuins as Sirtfoods.

Beyond antioxidants

To really understand the benefits of Sirtfoods requires us to think very differently about foods like fruits and vegetables, and the reasons they are good for us. There's absolutely no doubt that they are, with stacks of research testifying that diets rich in fruits, vegetables and plant foods generally slash the risk of many chronic diseases, including the biggest killers, heart disease and cancer. This has been put down to their rich content of nutrients, such as vitamins, minerals and of course, antioxidants, probably the biggest health buzzword of the last decade. But we're here to tell a very different story.

The reason Sirtfoods are so good for you has nothing to do with those nutrients we all know so well and hear so much about. Sure, they are all valuable things that you need to get from your diet, but there's something altogether different, and very special, going on with Sirtfoods. In fact, what if we threw that whole way of thinking on its head and said that the reason Sirtfoods are good for you is *not* because they nourish the body with essential nutrients, or provide antioxidants to mop up the damaging effects of free radicals, but quite the opposite; because they are full of weak toxins? In a world where almost every touted 'superfood' is aggressively marketed on the basis of its 'antioxidant' content, this might sound crazy. But it's a revolutionary idea, and one worth getting to grips with.

What doesn't kill you makes you stronger

Let's get back to the established ways of activating sirtuins for a moment: fasting and exercise. As we've seen, research has repeatedly shown that dietary energy restriction has dramatic benefits for weight loss, health and very possibly longevity. Then there's exercise, with its innumerable benefits for both body and mind, borne out by the finding that regular exercise dramatically slashes mortality rates[49]. But what is the one thing they all have in common?

The answer is: stress. They all cause a mild stress on the body that encourages it to adapt by becoming fitter, more efficient and more resilient. It's the body's response to these mildly stressful stimuli – its adaptation – that makes us fitter, healthier and leaner in the long run. And as we now know, these highly beneficial adaptations are orchestrated by sirtuins, which are switched on in the face of these stressors, and ignite a host of favourable changes in the body.

The technical term for adaptation to these stresses is hormesis. It's the idea that you get a beneficial effect from being exposed to a low dose of a substance or stress that is otherwise toxic or lethal if given at higher doses. Or, if you prefer, 'what doesn't kill you makes you stronger'. And that's exactly how fasting and exercise work. Starvation is lethal, and excessive exercise is detrimental to health. These extreme forms of stress are clearly harmful, but as long as they remain moderate and manageable stresses, they have highly beneficial effects.

Enter polyphenols

Now this is where things get truly fascinating. All living organisms experience hormesis, but what has been greatly underappreciated until now is that this also includes plants[50]. While we typically wouldn't think of plants as being the same as other living organisms, let alone a human, we actually share similar responses in terms of how we react, on a chemical level, to our environment.

As mind-blowing as that sounds, it makes perfect sense if we think about it in evolutionary terms, because all living things evolved to experience and cope with common environmental stresses such as dehydration, sunlight, nutrient deprivation and attack by pathogens.

If that is difficult to wrap your head around, get ready for the truly astonishing bit. Plant stress responses are actually more sophisticated than our own[51]. Think about it; if we are hungry and thirsty we can go in seek of food and drink; too hot – we find shade; under attack – we can flee. In complete contrast, plants are stationary, and as such, they must endure all the extremes of these physiological stresses and threats. In consequence, over the last billion years they have developed a highly sophisticated stress-response system that humbles anything we can boast. The way they do this is by producing a vast collection of natural plant chemicals – called polyphenols – that allow them to successfully adapt to their environment and survive. When we consume these plants, we also consume these polyphenol nutrients. Their effect is profound: they activate our own innate stress-response pathways. We're talking here about exactly the same pathways that fasting and exercise switch on; the sirtuins.

Piggybacking on a plant's stress-response system in this way, for our own benefit, is known as xenohormesis[52, 53]. And the implications are game-changing. Let the plants do the hard work so we don't have to. Indeed, these natural plant compounds are now referred to as caloric restriction mimetics due to their ability to turn on the same positive changes in our cells, such as fat burning, as would be seen during fasting[54, 55]. And by providing us with more advanced signalling compounds than we produce ourselves, the outcomes are superior to anything we can achieve through fasting or exercise alone.

> Due to a greater need to adapt to survive in their environment, foods grown in the wild, or even organically, are better for us than intensively farmed produce as they produce higher levels of polyphenols.

Sirtfoods

While all plants have these stress-response systems, only certain ones have developed to produce noteworthy amounts of sirtuin-activating polyphenols. We call these plants Sirtfoods. Their discovery means that instead of austere fasting regimes or arduous exercise programmes, there is now a revolutionary new way to activate your sirtuin genes: eating a diet abundant in Sirtfoods. Best of all, this one involves putting (Sirt)foods on to your plate, not taking them off!

It's so beautifully simple and so easy it seems like there must be a catch. But there isn't. This is how nature intended us to eat, rather than the stomach rumbling or calorie counting of modern dieting. Many of you who have experienced these hellish diets, where initial weight loss is fleeting before the body rebels and the weight comes piling back on, will understandably shudder at the thought of another false promise, another book boasting the dreaded 'D' word. But remember this: the modern approach to diet is only 150 years old; Sirtfoods were developed by nature over a billion years ago.

And with that you're probably itching to know what specific foods count as Sirtfoods. So without further ado, here are our top 20 Sirtfoods.

	Sirtfood	Major sirtuin-activating nutrients
1	Bird's-eye chilli	Luteolin, Myricetin
2	Buckwheat	Rutin
3	Capers	Kaempferol, Quercetin
4	Celery, including its leaves	Apigenin, Luteolin
5	Cocoa	Epicatechin
6	Coffee	Caffeic acid, Chlorogenic acid
7	Extra virgin olive oil	Oleuropein, Hydroxytyrosol
8	Green tea (especially matcha green tea)	Epigallocatechin gallate (EGCG)
9	Kale	Kaempferol, Quercetin
10	Lovage	Quercetin
11	Medjool dates	Gallic acid, Caffeic acid
12	Parsley	Apigenin, Myricetin
13	Red chicory	Luteolin
14	Red onion	Quercetin
15	Red wine	Resveratrol, Piceatannol
16	Rocket	Quercetin, Kaempferol
17	Soy	Daidzein, Formononetin
18	Strawberries	Fisetin
19	Turmeric	Curcumin
20	Walnuts	Gallic acid

SUMMARY

- We need to radically rethink the idea that fruits, vegetables and plant foods are good for us simply because they contain vitamins and antioxidants.

- Just like fasting and exercise, they are good for us because they contain natural chemicals that place a mild stress on our cells.

- Plants, because they are stationary, have developed a highly sophisticated stress-response system and produce polyphenols to help them adapt to the challenges of their environment.

- When we eat these plants, their polyphenols activate our stress-response pathways – our sirtuin genes – mimicking the effects of caloric restriction and exercise.

- The foods with the most powerful sirtuin-activating effects are called Sirtfoods.

Sirtfoods Around the World

You now know all about our ancient sirtuin genes, why they are so powerful and how they can be activated by Sirtfoods, but how does all of this play out in the real world?

Since ancient times, humans have been fascinated with the pursuit of the elixir of life. History is overcome with tales from ancient religions and myths where only gods and emperors were allowed to eat certain foods, foods which conferred power, strength and even immortality. Of course, this is the stuff of folklore, but with the discovery of Sirtfoods, for the first time ever, the realm of mythology has crossed over into reality.

Enter the Blue Zone

While our health is ailing, there are regions around the world, dubbed 'Blue Zones', where the intake of Sirtfoods is much, much higher than the amount we consume in a typical Western diet. Indeed, for the cultures eating Sirtfood-rich diets, the benefits seem more like the stuff of fantasy. In fact, not only do we see people living longer in Blue Zones than in countries where a typical Western diet is the norm, but much more important is how they retain youthful vitality in old age. In the Blue Zones, there are incredibly low rates of Alzheimer's, cancer, diabetes, heart disease and osteoporosis. Go there and you will see people aged 90 years of age or older walking, dancing and working. They are not active in the pursuit to lose weight, there's no need – there are no gyms. Instead they retain the vigour and energy of youth into old age. You will see them on motorcycles or riding bicycles in the street. Get chatting to them and you might hear them boast about how great their sex life still is! And it is of no surprise that they also happen to be the slimmest populations in the world.

I should cocoa

To better understand this incredible phenomenon, let's begin our journey with a trip to the San Blas islands of Panama and the indigenous home of the Kuna American Indians, who appear immune to high blood pressure and show remarkably low rates of obesity, diabetes, cancer and early death. At the turn of the twenty-first century a research team unearthed the Kuna's secret when they found that their major source of fluid was a beverage made from locally grown cocoa. This cocoa is fantastically rich in a specific group of polyphenols called flavanols, especially epicatechin, which qualifies it as a Sirtfood.

But how could we know that the rude health of the Kuna was down to their high intake of cocoa flavanols? The researchers found that when the Kuna Indians migrated to Panama City and switched to consuming intensively processed commercial cocoa (which is stripped of its flavanols and thus no longer a Sirtfood), the health benefits vanish[56].

The case of the Kuna is but one piece in a growing body of evidence that flavanol-rich cocoa has extraordinary health benefits. In clinical studies flavanol-rich cocoa has been found to improve blood pressure, blood flow, blood sugar control and cholesterol measures[57, 58]. Reviews suggest that cocoa also has positive effects in diabetes[59] and cancer[60]. And consumption has been shown to enhance memory performance, proffering a valuable dietary option in the search for the brain's fountain of youth[61].

Spice for life

Turmeric, known as 'Indian Solid Gold', has been used in Ayurvedic medicine for over 4,000 years for its wound-healing and anti-inflammatory properties. We now know these healing effects are down to the fact that it contains curcumin, a major sirtuin-activating nutrient, which makes it a Sirtfood.

It is a prevalent spice in traditional Indian cooking and is believed to contribute to the fact that cancer rates in India are significantly lower than in Western countries. Yet interestingly, the cancer rate for Indians increases by 50–75 per cent when they move from India to the USA and UK and abandon their traditional diet[62]. While this might be due to a number of different lifestyle factors, scientific evidence now indicates that curcumin has potent anti-cancer properties.

In addition to its anti-cancer claims there is mounting evidence of other sirtuin-activating health benefits. In recent studies, a special form of curcumin that was made to be more easily absorbed was shown to improve cholesterol levels, improve blood sugar control and reduce inflammation in the body[63]. It has been investigated for osteoarthritis of the knee and shown to be as effective as commonly taken painkillers[64]. And in patients with early type 2 diabetes, just eating a gram of turmeric a day improved their working memory[65].

The effectiveness of curcumin is limited because it is poorly absorbed by the body. However, research shows that by cooking it in liquid, adding fat, and adding black pepper we can dramatically increase its absorption. This fits perfectly with traditional Indian cooking, where it is typically combined with ghee and black pepper in curries and other hot dishes.

Green living

Green tea represents another tantalising Sirtfood offering. Green tea consumption is thought to have begun more than 4,700 years ago when the Chinese Emperor Shen Nung ('Divine Healer') produced a pleasant refreshing beverage with green tea leaves by serendipity. It was only much later that the beverage developed its reputation for medicinal and healing prowess.

Asia's high intake of green tea has been cited as a key reason for the 'Asian Paradox'. Despite an extremely high prevalence of cigarette smoking, Asia, and especially Japan, boasts some of the lowest rates of cardiovascular disease and lung cancer in the world. A high intake of green tea is linked with much lower rates of coronary heart disease and a reduced risk of many common cancers, such as those affecting the prostate, stomach, lung and breast. It is little wonder therefore that green tea consumption is linked to substantially fewer early deaths.

Intriguingly, green tea also has a thermogenic effect, which means it increases the amount of energy the body burns off, aiding fat loss while maintaining muscle. Combine green tea with a diet abundant in leafy greens, soy, herbs and spices (turmeric use is especially prevalent), to create a smorgasbord of Sirtfoods, and we have a diet very similar to that found in Okinawa – 'the land of the immortals'.

Okinawa might be the poorest province in Japan, yet it holds the record for longevity and the greatest number of centenarians in the world. So astounding is their quality of life, researchers assumed it must be down to superior genes. But, along came the 'Westernisation' of its diet and with it burgeoning rates of obesity and crippling diseases that younger generations are now experiencing for the first time, firmly putting any idea of superior genes to rest.

A Mediterranean prescription

For a true bounty of Sirtfood combinations, we need to travel to the Mediterranean. This is where we find regular consumption of a host of potent Sirtfoods – extra virgin olive oil, nuts, berries, green leafy vegetables, herbs and spices, and of course, wine. Eating this type of diet is linked to a 9 per cent reduction in death from all causes, with substantial reductions in cardiovascular disease and degenerative brain diseases like Alzheimer's, as well as cancer[66].

A landmark trial of the Mediterranean diet called Predimed was carried out in Spain on almost 7,400 individuals at high risk of cardiovascular disease. The results were so good that the trial was stopped early, after five years. People who were encouraged to deliberately focus on eating extra Sirtfoods (especially extra virgin olive oil and nuts – predominantly walnuts) experienced incredible results, reducing their incidence of cardiovascular disease by approximately 30 per cent[67] – a result that drug manufacturers can only dream about. Offshoots of the study showed a 30 per cent reduction in diabetes too[68], as well as significant drops in levels of inflammation[69] and improvements in memory and overall brain health[70].

Researchers also did something very interesting. They examined the genetic profile for PPAR-γ – which, if you remember, is the obesity villain we came across earlier. While some of us are quite resistant to its actions, others are not so fortunate, and can get really clobbered by it. This means you might eat the same as someone else but be much more susceptible to weight gain. However, it doesn't need to be that way with Sirtfoods. In those who followed the Sirtfood-rich Mediterranean diet, the negative effects of this gene were reversed[71]. Incredibly, despite no drop in calories, the diet richer in Sirtfoods was linked to a 40 per cent drop in the risk of obesity, especially weight stored around the tummy[72]. Forget low fat and forget obsessing over calories: those who follow a traditional Mediterranean diet will always be slimmer than the general population.

So there we have it. The cultures around the world who are healthiest, slimmest and live the longest lives have something in common: they eat the highest amount of Sirtfoods. They stay lean and slim without so much as counting a calorie or going on a diet. That leaves us to do just one thing, which is to piece together all of the most potent

Sirtfoods on the planet to create a diet the likes of which has never been seen before. In essence, a diet to drive a health and weight-loss revolution.

SUMMARY

- While obesity and chronic disease are rampant in the Western world, there are 'Blue Zones' that are virtually immune from these problems.

- One thing that people living in Blue Zones have in common is a diet very rich in Sirtfoods.

- Classic examples include the Kuna American Indians and their penchant for cocoa, the turmeric-infused diet of India, the Japanese predilection for green tea and the extra virgin olive oil at the heart of the traditional Mediterranean diet.

- *The Sirtfood Diet* brings together all these great foods – and more – into a world-beating diet for health and weight loss.

7

The Sirtfood Diet

By now you know all about sirtuins, how they help us burn fat, maintain muscle and promote exceptional health. You will also have learnt about Sirtfoods, how they can switch on our sirtuin genes, and how they form the basis for the diets of the healthiest and longest-living populations on the planet. And here we are ready to kick off on a journey to a slimmer, leaner and healthier you. So let us get started by guiding you through the Sirtfood Diet and how it works.

The best of the best

With the Sirtfood Diet we have done something very special. We've taken the most potent Sirtfoods on the planet and have woven them into a brand-new way of eating, the likes of which has never been seen before. We have selected the 'best of the best' from the healthiest diets ever known and from them created a world-beating diet.

The good news is, you don't have to suddenly adopt the traditional diet of an Okinawan or be able to cook like an Italian mamma. That's not only completely unrealistic, but totally unnecessary on the Sirtfood Diet. Indeed, one thing that may strike you from the list of Sirtfoods (see page 56) is their familiarity. While you may not currently be eating all the foods on the list you most likely are consuming some. So why are you not already losing weight?

The answer can be found when we examine both the quantity and the variety needed to get results.

Hitting your quota

Right now, most people simply don't consume nearly enough Sirtfoods to illicit a potent fat-burning and health-boosting effect. When researchers looked at consumption of five key sirtuin-activating nutrients (quercetin, myricetin, kaempferol, luteolin and apigenin) in the US diet they found individual daily intakes to be a miserly 13mg per day[73]. In contrast the average Japanese intake was five times higher[74]. Compare that with our Sirtfood Diet trial, where individuals were consuming hundreds of milligrams of sirtuin-activating nutrients every day.

What we are talking about is a total diet revolution where

we increase our daily intake of sirtuin-activating nutrients by as much as 50-fold. While this may sound daunting or impractical, it really isn't. By taking all our top Sirtfoods and putting them together in a way that is totally compatible with your busy life, you too can easily and effectively reach the level of intake needed to reap all the benefits.

Plants vs pharmaceuticals

One question you may rightly ask is: why can't I just take a pill to reach these quantities? After all, the pharmaceutical industry is perfectly aware that sirtuins are a treasure chest waiting to be opened, if only they could find the right key. They've already invested hundreds of millions in trying to do just that, either extracting the active components from Sirtfoods, most famously resveratrol, from the skin of grapes, or developing man-made synthetic molecules aimed at activating sirtuins. However, results to date have been underwhelming, which in fact, should be in no way surprising.

When it comes to diet, there are two options. One is to take advantage of nature and what it has developed in harmony with mankind; the other is to rise above our station and think we can hijack nature and better it. The latter has been tried many times, which involves isolating a single compound and prescribing it in pharmacological doses. This is exactly the approach that all too often gives rise to unwanted or unforeseen side effects that are the Achilles heel of so many pharmaceutical drugs and for that matter many nutritional supplements.

THE POWER OF SYNERGY

We believe it is better to consume a wide range of these wonder nutrients in the form of natural wholefoods, where they co-exist alongside the hundreds of other natural bio-active plant chemicals which act synergistically to boost our health. We think it is better to work with nature, rather than against it.

Take for example the classic sirtuin-activating nutrient resveratrol. In supplement form it is poorly absorbed, but in its natural food matrix of red wine, its bioavailability (how much the body can use) is at least six-fold higher[75, 76]. Add to this the fact that red wine contains not just one, but a whole range of polyphenols, which act together to bring health benefits, including the sirtuin activator piceatannol. While rarely receiving the limelight, researchers are now beginning to realise piceatannol has important health benefits in its own right. It's not difficult to see why isolating a single nutrient is nowhere near as effective as consuming it in its whole food form.

But what makes a dietary approach really special is when we begin to combine multiple Sirtfoods. For example, by adding in quercetin-rich Sirtfoods we enhance the bioavailability of resveratrol-containing foods even further. Not only this, but their actions complement each other. Both are fat busters, but there are nuances in how each of them achieves this. Resveratrol is very effective at helping to destroy existing fat cells, whereas quercetin excels in preventing new fat cell formation[77]. In combination we are targeting fat from both sides resulting in a greater impact on fat loss than if we just ate large amounts of a single food.

And this is a pattern we see over and again. Foods rich in the sirtuin activator apigenin improve the absorption of quercetin from food, and enhance its activity[78]. In turn, quercetin has been shown to synergise with the activity of epigallocatechin gallate (EGCG)[79]. And EGCG has been shown to work synergistically with curcumin[80]. And so it goes on. Not only are individual whole foods more potent than isolated nutrients, but by combining Sirtfoods we tap into a whole tapestry of health benefits that nature has weaved – so intricate, so refined, it is impossible to try and trump it.

Additionally, while we have based the Sirtfood Diet around the 20 foods with the highest levels of sirtuin-activating compounds to deliver the maximum weight loss and health benefits, there are many other healthy foods that we encourage you to eat too. The beauty of this is that some of them actually powerfully enhance the effect of our chosen Sirtfoods.

For example, a building block of dietary protein, called leucine, has been shown to work synergistically with the wonder nutrients found in Sirtfoods to amplify their beneficial effects[81, 82]. This is why we base many of our meals around not just Sirtfoods, but also protein-rich foods, in order to deliver the right quantity of leucine to increase their effectiveness.

Likewise, you will undoubtedly have heard lots about the health benefits of oily fish and specifically omega-3 fish oils. Recent research has shown that omega-3 fish oils can favourably influence the way our sirtuin genes work too[83]. This helps us to further understand why fish oils are good for us and adds yet another dimension to the food we have at our disposal to enhance the effect of a sirtuin-activating diet. By tapping into this incredible synergy, you can begin to see just how powerful the Sirtfood Diet is.

A taste revolution

A fundamental problem with conventional dieting is that it typically makes for a miserable dining experience. It drains every last drop of pleasure from food leaving us feeling dissatisfied. But for us, it's essential that you maintain the joy of food in the pursuit of a healthy weight. That's why we were delighted when we realised that Sirtfoods, as well as the foods that enhance their actions, i.e. protein and omega-3 food sources, are primed to satisfy our desire for taste. It's the ultimate win-win: the Sirtfood Diet boosts our health *and* tastes great.

Let's take a step back to see how this occurs. Our taste buds determine how tasty we find our food, and how satisfied we are from eating it. This is done through seven major taste receptors. Over countless generations, humans have evolved to seek out the tastes that stimulate these receptors in order to achieve maximum nourishment from our diet. The better a food stimulates these taste receptors, the more satisfaction we get from a meal. And in the Sirtfood Diet we have the ultimate menu for happy taste buds as it offers maximum stimulation across all taste receptors. To summarise these tastes and the foods you'll be eating on the diet that satisfy them – the seven major taste sensations are sweet (strawberries, dates); salty (celery, fish); sour (strawberries); bitter (cocoa, kale, chicory, extra virgin olive oil, green tea); pungent (chillies, extra virgin olive oil), astringent (green tea, red wine) and umami (soy, fish, meat).

Crucially, what we have discovered is that the greater the sirtuin-activating properties of a food, the more powerfully it stimulates those taste centres, and the more gratification we get from the food we eat. Importantly, it also means that we satisfy our appetite quicker, and our desire to eat more is reduced accordingly. This is a key reason why those who follow a Sirtfood-rich diet are pleasantly fuller more quickly.

For example, natural cocoa has a striking bitter flavour, but remove the sirtuin-activating flavanols with aggressive industrial food-processing techniques and we are left with mass-produced, bland and characterless cocoa that is used to make highly sugared chocolate confectionary. By this point, the health benefits have vanished.

The same principle applies to olive oil. Consumed in its minimally processed form – extra virgin – it has a powerful and distinct flavour, with an invigorating kick that can be felt at the back of the throat. Yet refined and processed olive oil loses all character, is mild and bland and carries no such kick. Similarly, bird's eye chillies boast much greater sirtuin-activating credentials than the milder standard chillies that are more commonly used, and wild strawberries are much tastier than farmed ones due to a richer content of sirtuin-activating nutrients.

Not only this, we also find that individual Sirtfoods can trigger multiple taste receptors: green tea is both bitter and astringent and strawberries have a combination of sweet and sour flavours.

GOOD TASTE

While you may not be so used to some of these flavours, you can acquire a taste for them very rapidly and grow to appreciate and love them. For example, we know many people who once they get accustomed to the complex flavours in dark chocolate with a high percentage of cocoa solids would never dream about switching back to the sugary confectionary version. You can now even find dark chocolate that comes with tasting notes, just like a good wine! Of course we don't need to go that far, but what you will discover is that eating Sirtfoods in their natural form provides ample thrills and delights for your palate.

What all this means is that humans evolved to seek out a diet rich in Sirtfoods, alongside healthful protein and omega-3 fatty acids, to satisfy the basic desires of our appetite, and in turn, our health. This evolutionary process occurred over millennia, without us knowing the reasons, yet it ensured we got maximum benefit from consuming these foods.

Sadly, fast forward to the present day, and we no longer eat enough of these natural foods that genuinely satisfy our appetite. Instead we have resorted to 'empty' industrialised food, in which overwhelming amounts of salt or sugar are added during the processing and which ultimately fail to truly satisfy us – a reason we end up overconsuming them. But by getting back to Sirtfoods we spark a gastronomic revolution whereby eating a combination of Sirtfoods is the ultimate natural appetite satisfier.

A DIET OF INCLUSION

Let's try an experiment. We just want you to do one really simple thing for us: don't think of a white bear . . .

What did you just think of? A white bear, of course. Why? Because we told you not to. Don't tell us you are still thinking about it!

This was the trailblazing experiment performed by

psychology professor Daniel Wegner in 1987, which showed that forced suppression of thoughts causes a paradoxical and counterproductive escalation in how often we actually think about what we are trying to suppress[84]. So instead of blocking it from our thoughts it produces a preoccupation with the suppressed thought.

And as you've probably guessed this phenomenon is not just applicable to white bears. The exact same thing happens when we make villains of and restrict foods for weight loss. Studies show we actually think about them more often, increasing temptation. It eats away at us until we eat it! And with the diet broken and the escalated thinking about the 'forbidden' foods we endured, we are now much more likely to binge.

Scientists have now explained what is happening here. We all have a deep need to be autonomous. When we feel controlled, such as going on a strict diet, it creates a negative environment that makes us feel uneasy. We feel captives of this negativity and rebel to break out of it. We rebel by doing what we were told we should not, and doing it a lot more than we would have in the first place. It happens to all of us, even the most self-controlled. It's not a matter of if, but when. Scientists now believe this is a critical reason why we can maintain diets and even see results in the initial stages but fail to see long-term success.

So does this mean there is no point in even attempting to change our eating habits? Are we just destined for failure?

No, it means that when we make change, in order to succeed we need to make it our own positive, desired decision. We now know the way to achieve this is not through dietary *exclusion* but through dietary *inclusion*. Rather than focusing your energy on the negatives of what you should not be eating, instead you focus on the positives of what you should be eating. By doing this you avoid the psychological backlash. And this is the beauty of the Sirtfood Diet. It's about what you put into your diet, not what you take out. It's about the *quality* of your food not the *quantity*. And it's about you wanting to do it because you feel satisfied by eating great-tasting foods with the added knowledge each bite provides a bounty of benefits.

Most diets are a means to an end. It's about hanging in there, trying to keep sight of the 'thin ideal'. But ultimately it rarely comes before the diet fails, and even if it is achieved, it's rarely sustained. The Sirtfood Diet is different. It is all about the journey. Phase 1, which does restrict calories, is kept purposely short and sweet to ensure it is finished with motivating results before any negative backlash. Then the focus is solely about Sirtfoods. And the motivation for eating Sirtfoods is not driven just by an end result of weight loss. Instead it is as much if not more about the appreciation and enjoyment of real food for a healthy and fit lifestyle.

What's more, once you are reaping the unique benefits of Sirtfoods, from satisfying your appetite to increasing your quality of life, you will find that your habits and tastes change.

With the Sirtfood Diet, foods that would previously have set off the cascade of negative reactions if you were told you could not eat them will lose their appeal and their hold over you will diminish. They become a minor part of your diet, and all achieved without a single sighting of a white bear.

SUMMARY

- The Sirtfood Diet takes the most potent Sirtfoods on the planet and brings them together in a simple and practical way of eating.

- We focus on whole foods not isolated supplements or drugs to deliver a rich synergy of sirtuin-activating compounds.

- We further enhance this by including other healthy ingredients, such as leucine-rich protein foods and oily fish, to make the effects of the Sirtfood Diet even more powerful.

- Unlike our modern diets, Sirtfoods satisfy all our taste receptors which means we get more gratification from our food and feel content quicker.

- The Sirtfood Diet is a diet of inclusion – not exclusion, making it the only type of diet that can deliver long-term weight-loss success.

8

Phase 1: 7lb in Seven Days

Starting on the road to weight-loss success and better health begins with Phase 1 of the Sirtfood Diet. This is what we like to call the hyper-success phase, where you will take a huge step towards achieving the slimmer and leaner body you want with our clinically proven method for losing 7lb (3.2kg) in seven days. This will be achieved by powerfully combining moderate fasting with a specially designed diet very rich in Sirtfoods. Follow our simple step-by-step instructions and make use of the delicious recipes provided for you. As well as our standard 7-day plan, we also have a meat-free version, which is suitable for both vegetarians and vegans. Feel free to go with whichever one you prefer.

What to expect

If you are like the majority of people who have followed Phase 1, you can expect to lose somewhere in the region of 7lb (3.2kg) during this phase. But remember this also includes muscle gain, so don't be disappointed if your number falls a bit short (see page 12). The numbers on the scales won't necessarily tell you the whole story. As we have clearly seen, for both men and women alike, it is much more desirable to lose fat with an accompanying gain in muscle, instead of just looking for the biggest possible drop in weight. The bathroom scales are one way to measure your progress, but it won't necessarily give you the full story of how much fat you have lost and how your body composition has improved. So what are others?

Rather than relying solely on scales, we encourage you to look out for other signs that your body composition is transforming. Ask yourself, how are your clothes fitting? Are your trousers looser around the waist? Or better still, wait for the compliments you'll receive from your friends and family about how slim and toned you suddenly look . . .

It is also important not to get too caught up with your expectation of how much weight you will lose at the end of the seven days. We know that those who focus too much on the expected outcome, instead of spending their time engaging positively with the process itself, are less successful. One of the reasons we believe our trial was so successful is because no one went into it expecting to achieve those weight-loss results. When we began the trial, we expected some weight loss, but never anticipated that the results in this relatively fit and healthy population would be 7lb (3.2kg). Most participants were not even classed as over-weight to begin with. The reason they did it was for all the health and well-being benefits that combining Sirtfoods with mild fasting brings. They freely chose to embark on the 7-day plan, motivated by the desire for a fitter and healthier body.

Just like them, we encourage you to put equal emphasis on measuring other outcomes such as changes in your sense of well-being, your energy levels and how clear your skin looks. You can even get measurements of your overall cardiovascular and metabolic health performed at your local pharmacy to see changes in things like your blood pressure, blood sugar levels, and blood fats such as choles-terol and triglycerides.

But most of all we encourage you to positively engage in and enjoy the process. Throughout the seven days, you will experience the power of Sirtfoods, and with this you will also learn lots of interesting facts about the foods you are eating and why they are so good for you.

Above all, we want you to appreciate that the Sirtfood Diet is not just a means to an end but the foundation for a future of a slimmer and healthier you. One where you cannot only sustain those benefits but develop a more positive relationship with the food you eat, by knowing the power of inclusion over exclusion.

Phase 1

Phase 1 of the Sirtfood Diet is based on two distinct stages:

Days 1–3 are the most intensive and during this period you can eat up to a limit of 1,000 calories each day, consisting of:

- 3 x Sirtfood green juices
- 1 x main meal

Days 4–7 will see your food intake increase to a limit of 1,500 calories each day, consisting of:

- 2 x Sirtfood green juices
- 2 x main meals

The use of juices and whole food is an integral part of the Sirtfood Diet. Juices give maximum bang for your buck by packing in a super-concentrated amount of Sirtfoods into an ultra-easy and convenient way to consume them. Having some of your Sirtfoods in the form of a juice can also have big advantages when it comes to absorbing their goodness. For example, one of the ingredients we include in the green juice is matcha green tea. When we consume the sirtuin activator EGCG, found in high levels in green tea, in drink form without food its absorption is more than 65 per cent higher[85].

Yet eating whole food has definite advantages too. Many Sirtfoods contain significant amounts of what are called non-extractable polyphenols (or NEPPs). These are polyphenols, including sirtuin activators, which are attached to the fibrous part of the food, and are only released when broken down by our friendly gut bacteria. As juicing removes the fibre from our food, if we relied on it alone, we would lose out on all those valuable NEPPs.

The key is to get the best of both worlds by combining the two. Vegetables like leafy greens have low levels of NEPPs so are much more suitable for concentrating through juicing, whereas other higher fibre Sirtfoods are more appropriate for eating whole and enjoying as part of your meals.

There are few rules for when you have to consume the juices and meals. Ultimately their consumption needs to fit in with your day-to-day life, however, a few simple rules of thumb for the best outcome are:

- It's better to spread the juices out throughout the day, rather than having them too close together.
- The green juices should be consumed at least an hour before or two hours after meals.
- Meals or juices should not be consumed later than 7pm.

The reason we recommend you do not eat past 7pm is to keep eating habits in tune with your internal body clock. We all have an in-built body clock, called our circadian rhythm, which regulates many of our natural body functions according to the time of the day. Among other things, this influences how the body handles the food we eat. And studies show that when food is consumed early in the day we are most likely to use it for energy, whereas if we eat late in the day the food is processed differently, being more likely to be stored as fat. This makes sense because early in the day is the time when we are usually active and require energy. But later in the day, the body gears up for rest and sleep and lowers its energy demands. It's called your body-fat clock and eating in tune with it will help you get better results. In fact, evidence now suggests that sirtuin activation actually enhances this circadian rhythm[86], which means that by eating Sirtfoods early in the day we can prime our natural body-fat clock and rev up energy burning during this period even more effectively.

BE GUIDED BY YOUR APPETITE

One of the surprising things we observed is that people following the seven-day plan didn't report feeling as hungry as we expected. In fact, it was much more common to hear that people couldn't actually eat all the food that was given to them and ended up almost forcing it down!

We don't want you to do that. Our advice is to prepare the meals as per the instructions but then just eat them according to your appetite. If you're hungry and devour all of it, that's fine, but if you find you are comfortably full, then stop, even if that means leaving some of the food you have prepared.

WHAT TO DRINK

As well as the recommended daily servings of green juices, you can consume other fluids freely throughout Phase 1. These should be non-caloric drinks, preferably plain water, black coffee and green tea.

Many people have been surprised that not only do we allow black coffee during this phase of the diet, but that we actively encourage it. Remember, coffee is a Sirtfood and contrary to the popular belief that coffee is bad for you, considerable research now shows that drinking coffee is linked with numerous health benefits. We recommend that coffee be drunk black, without adding milk, as some researchers have found that the addition of milk can reduce the absorption of the beneficial sirtuin-activating nutrients[87]. The same has been found for green tea[88], though adding some lemon juice actually increases the absorption of its sirtuin-activating nutrients[89].

The only thing to be aware of is that we do not recommend a big change to your normal coffee consumption.

Caffeine withdrawal symptoms can make you feel lousy for a couple of days; likewise, large increases can be unpleasant in those particularly sensitive to the effects of caffeine.

We are also aware that the UK is a nation divided, and if you are not a coffee drinker there's a high chance you have a preference for tea. If that's what you enjoy we won't get in your way and black tea is perfectly fine to include (even if you take it with a dash of milk). Likewise, some people prefer white tea, a very close relation to green tea.

Do remember that this is the hyper-success phase and while you should be comforted by the fact that it is for one week only, you do need to be a bit more disciplined. For this week we only include alcohol as a cooking ingredient. And with plenty of green juices to consume, and a whole world of Sirtfoods to explore, we leave soft drinks and fruit juices behind. If you do get a hankering for these, use this week as an opportunity to try adding some sliced strawberries to still or sparkling water, to make your own Sirtfood-infused water. Keep it in the fridge for a couple of hours and you'll have a pleasantly refreshing alternative to soft drinks and juices. Any combination of lemon, lime, cucumber, mint and basil also make great additions for more variety of tastes and to keep it interesting. Enjoy experimenting to find which combinations work best for you.

What do I need to get started?

The one piece of kit you need to follow the Sirtfood Diet is a juicer to make the essential daily green juices. While there is a lot of talk about different types of juicers and which is best, we're not too hung up on that. If you don't already own one, just get one that fits within your budget.

ARE ALL THE FOODS EASY TO GET?

Virtually all of our top 20 Sirtfoods (see page 56) will be very familiar to you and are readily available, whether that be at your local supermarket, market or farm shop. But there are some exceptions.

The first is matcha, which is an essential ingredient in the green juices. Matcha is a powdered green tea and is widely available online, from health-food stores and is also starting to appear in supermarkets. There can be quite a large variance in price, and some brands are expensive, so do shop around. Matcha will typically come from Japan or China. As matcha from China is known to be at high risk of contamination, especially with lead, from China's highly polluted atmosphere (and this includes organic varieties), we recommend you buy Japanese brands.

The second of our less well-known Sirtfoods is the sadly overlooked culinary herb lovage. The good news is, it's really easy to grow yourself. All you need is a few seeds, a tray or a pot and windowsill to place it on. Or easier still if you get down to your local garden centre and buy a pot of growing lovage and grow it on yourself. You will also find online stockists of both lovage seeds and plants. While we're big fans of lovage and would love to see its renaissance, we appreciate it requires you to go the extra mile, and we don't want that to prevent you getting started. We do encourage you to include it in your diet but don't worry if you can't, as you'll still experience the multitude of benefits from all the other Sirtfoods.

Last is buckwheat. The reason that buckwheat is head and shoulders above other more common grains is probably due to the fact that it is not a grain at all. It would be more apt to refer to it as a 'pseudo-grain'. A wonderful carbohydrate and protein source, as well as a Sirtfood powerhouse, it makes a great alternative to more commonly used grains, even though it is actually a fruit seed related to rhubarb. Buckwheat groats are available in most supermarkets, and they continue to grow in popularity. However, the puffs, flakes and pasta are easiest sourced at a local health store or at online retailers. Our recipes also include buckwheat noodles (known as soba). These are available in supermarkets but you will need to check the packet carefully as they are often made from a combination of buckwheat and wheat. For those who want maximum benefit or those who need to avoid gluten, you need to seek out 100 per cent buckwheat noodles, again from health-food shops or online retailers.

The Sirtfood green juice

The green juice is an essential part of Phase 1 of the Sirtfood Diet. All the ingredients are powerful Sirtfoods, and in each juice you get a potent cocktail of natural compounds such as apigenin, kaempferol, luteolin, quercetin, and EGCG, that work together to switch on your sirtuin genes and promote fat loss. All we've added to that is a touch of apple for taste, and some lemon. Don't overlook the lemon. Its natural acidity has been shown to protect, stabilise and increase the absorption of the drink's sirtuin-activating nutrients.

You will get to know this green juice well, so, what are the ingredients you will be using?

- Kale
- Rocket
- Parsley
- Lovage (optional)
- Green celery, including its leaves
- Matcha green tea

KALE

We are cynics at heart so we are always sceptical of what's driving the latest 'superfood' publicity craze. Is it science or is it vested interests? Few foods have exploded on the health scene in recent years as ferociously as kale. Described as the 'lean, green, brassica queen' it has become the chic vegetable all health enthusiasts and foodies are gunning for. There is even a National Kale Day organised each October. But you don't have to wait until then to show your kale pride, there are T-shirts too, with trendy slogans such as 'Powered by Kale' and 'Highway to Kale'. For us, that's enough to set the alarm bells ringing. Filled with suspicions, we did the research, and we have to admit our conclusion is that it does actually deserve its plaudits (although we still don't recommend the T-shirt!). The reason we are pro-kale is that it boasts bumper amounts of the sirtuin-activating nutrients quercetin and kaempferol, making it a must-include in any diet and the base of our Sirtfood green juice. What's so refreshing about kale is that unlike the usual exotic, difficult-to-source and exorbitantly priced so-called 'superfoods', it is available everywhere, grows locally here in the UK and is very affordable.

ROCKET

Next into the juicer is rocket, a leafy green with a long and interesting history. It was first cultivated in Ancient Rome where it was revered for being a potent aphrodisiac. It then became extremely popular across Europe, including Britain, in the Middle Ages but went out of fashion as eating habits changed with the ushering in of Victorian

Britain. It is very aromatic and has a distinct peppery taste. In addition to its use in the green juice, its fantastic flavour, along with its potent sirtuin-activating nutrients, makes it our leaf of choice for all salad bases, where it pairs perfectly with an extra virgin olive oil dressing. Rocket is widely available as two distinct types: salad rocket (also known as arugula) and wild rocket. It doesn't matter which one you use as both are excellent Sirtfoods – and both equally delicious.

PARSLEY

Parsley is a culinary conundrum. It appears so often in recipes, yet so often it's the token green guy. At best we serve a few sprigs chopped up and tossed on a meal as an afterthought, at worst a solitary sprig purely for decorative purposes. Either way, it's often still languishing there on the plate long after we've finished eating. This typecasting stems from its traditional use in Ancient Rome as a garnish to eat after meals to refresh breath, instead of being part of the meal itself. And what a shame because parsley is a fantastic food packing a vibrant and refreshing taste that's filled with character. Taste aside, what makes parsley really special is that it is an excellent source of the sirtuin-activating nutrient apigenin, which is rarely found in significant quantities in other foods. Instead of its current ubiquitous use as food confetti, it's time we appreciated parsley as a food in its own right, along with the wonderful health benefits it can bring.

LOVAGE

Lovage is one of the world's oldest culinary herbs and at one time was among the most popular used. It is an extremely versatile plant possessing flavours of both celery and parsley, but much stronger, as well as having aromatic undertones for an intriguing taste. Just like rocket it was considered an aphrodisiac and Charlemagne (Charles the Great) had all his gardens planted in 'love parsley'. It is said that it was brought to Britain by the Romans, where it was rapidly accepted as a firm culinary favourite. Sadly, this delicious and once staple British salad green has now fallen off our gastronomic radars. But don't fear, as we're feeling the love for lovage once more, and want to see its resurrection as a staple on our plates and in our herb gardens. That's because it is not just delicious but also an extraordinarily rich source of the sirtuin-activating compound quercetin. So rather than just give up on this wonderful but long-lost indigenous culinary herb, it's time it had its renaissance in our diet.

CELERY

Celery has been around for millennia, but as early strains were very bitter it was usually regarded as a medicinal plant. As sweeter varieties developed it gained notoriety as an edible plant and took off in Britain in the Victorian era, where it became established as a traditional salad vegetable. When it comes to celery it is important to note there are two types: blanched/yellow and Pascal/green. Blanching is a technique that was developed to reduce celery's characteristic taste, which was perceived to be too strong. What a travesty that is for as well as dumbing down the flavour, blanching also dumbs down its sirtuin-activating properties. Luckily the tide is changing and people are demanding real and distinct flavour and are turning back to the more vivid green variety. Green celery is available in all good supermarkets now, and is the type we recommend that you use in the green juices and meals, with the most nutritious parts being the hearts and the leaves.

MATCHA GREEN TEA

Think of matcha as normal green tea on steroids. It is a special powdered green tea treasured by the Japanese and used in the traditional Zen monk Japanese tea ceremony (Sadō) which became extremely popular with the samurai, royalty and Japan's upper class. As described by a Zen priest in the eleventh century '(matcha) tea is the ultimate mental and medical remedy and has the ability to make one's life more full and complete.'

Matcha is grown in 90 per cent shade, while common green tea is usually grown in bright sunlight. Matcha leaves are then ground to a fine powder using a stone mill. In contrast to common green tea, which is drunk as an infusion, when matcha is consumed, the finely ground leaves themselves are dissolved into water and ingested. The upshot of consuming matcha in this way is that it results in dramatically greater intakes of the sirt-activating compound EGCG compared with other types of green tea.

Sirtfood green juice (serves 1)

2 large handfuls (75g) kale
a large handful (30g) rocket
a very small handful (5g) flat-leaf parsley
a very small handful (5g) lovage leaves (optional)
2–3 large stalks (150g) green celery, including its leaves
½ medium green apple
juice of ½ lemon
½ level tsp matcha*

Note that while in our pilot trial all quantities were weighed out exactly as listed, our experience is that handful measures work extremely well. In fact they better tailor the

* Phase1 – days 1–3: added to the first two juices of the day only; days 4–7: added to both juices

nutrient quantity to an individual's body size. Larger individuals tend to have larger hands and therefore get a proportionally higher amount of Sirtfood nutrients to match their body size and vice versa for smaller people.

- Mix the greens (kale, rocket, parsley and lovage, if using) together, then juice them. We find juicers can really differ in their efficiency at juicing leafy vegetables and you may need to re-juice the remnants before moving on to the other ingredients. The goal is to end up with about 50ml of juice from the greens.
- Now juice the celery and apple.
- You can peel the lemon and put it through the juicer as well, but we find it much easier to simply squeeze the lemon by hand into the juice. By this stage, you should have around 250ml of juice in total, perhaps slightly more.
- It is only when the juice is made and ready to serve that you add the matcha. Pour a small amount of the juice into a glass, then add the matcha and stir vigorously with a fork or teaspoon. We only use matcha in the first two drinks of the day as it contains moderate amounts of caffeine (the same content as a normal cup of tea). For people not used to it, it may keep them awake if drunk late.
- Once the matcha is dissolved add the remainder of the juice. Give it a final stir, then your juice is ready

to drink. Feel free to top up with plain water,
according to taste.

You can either make each juice from scratch when you want it, or you can make up all your juices for the day in one batch in the morning, and refrigerate until needed, without any loss of potency. In fact research points to the beneficial sirtuin-activating polyphenols lasting for up to three days before levels start to drop, so if you're short on time it's perfectly fine to make your juices for the day in advance, ensuring you keep them chilled and away from light.

Phase 1: your 7-day guide

DAY 1

Today welcomes the beginning (Please note that you need to read the recipe notes on page 170 before cooking.)of your new and exciting journey on the Sirtfood Diet.

We begin this week's meals with a delicious stir-fry that is super-quick and easy but has full-on flavour. It's not just their convenience or the fact that they are brimming with Sirtfoods that make stir-fries a stellar choice; they are actually a very favourable method of preparing food to retain the powerful sirtuin-activating goodness of the ingredients. Take red onions, which we have included because they are chock-full of quercetin. Red onions come up trumps with the highest quercetin content but the standard yellow ones don't lag too far behind. Onions lose 20 per cent of their quercetin content when fried, but this jumps to 65 per cent when microwaved and a truly disappointing loss of 75 per cent when boiled[90]. So, not only does stir-frying lock in loads of flavour, but also lots of the sirtuin-activating polyphenols.

Today we also introduce you to buckwheat. Extremely popular in Japan, the story goes that when Buddhist monks made long trips into the mountains all they would bring was a cooking pot and a bag of buckwheat for food. So nutritious is buckwheat that this was all they needed, and it nourished them for weeks. As you will see over the coming days, we are big buckwheat fans, and that's down to the fact that it is one of the best-known sources of a sirtuin activator called rutin. It's as versatile as any grain going, and being naturally gluten-free it is also a great choice for those who are gluten intolerant.

On day 1, you will consume:

- 3 x Sirtfood green juice (pages 93–5)
- 1 x main meal (either standard or vegan option, see below)

Take the juices at separate times of the day (e.g. first thing in the morning, mid-morning and mid-afternoon) and select one of the standard or vegan meal options:

Asian king prawn stir-fry with buckwheat
noodles (pages 172–3)

+

15–20g dark chocolate
(85 per cent cocoa solids; see Day 2 below)

or

Miso and sesame glazed tofu with ginger and
chilli stir-fried greens (vegan, pages 174–5)

+

15–20g dark chocolate (85 per cent cocoa solids)

DAY 2

Welcome aboard day 2. The formula stays the same as for day 1 and the only thing that changes is your main meal. Today you will see dark chocolate repeating itself on the menu, as it will again tomorrow. Simply put, for this wonder food, we really don't need an excuse to eat it. In chapter 6 we saw the amazing health benefits that cocoa possesses, and for the last four millennia we have had a love affair with this delicious Sirtfood.

In ancient civilisations, such as the Aztecs and Mayans, cocoa was considered a sacred food and usually reserved for the elite and the warriors, being served at feasts to gain loyalty and obligation. Indeed, the cocoa bean was held in such high regard that it was even used as a form of currency.

Back then it was usually served as a frothy drink. But what could be a more delicious way of getting our dietary cocoa quota than through chocolate?

Alas, the diluted, refined and highly sweetened milk chocolate we commonly munch doesn't count here. To earn its Sirtfood badge we are talking about chocolate with 85 per cent cocoa solids. But even then, cocoa percentage aside, not all chocolate is created equal. Chocolate is often treated with an alkalising agent (known as 'Dutch process') to reduce its acidity and give it a darker colour. Sadly, this process massively diminishes its sirtuin-activating flavanols, thus seriously compromising its health-promoting qualities. While in the USA these products are clearly labelled 'processed with alkali', unfortunately no such labelling requirement exists in the UK, making it difficult to know which brand to choose to reap the true benefits of cocoa. Well, we're pleased to share the fruits of our investigations and reveal that Lindt Excellence 85% Cocoa bar is confirmed as not having undergone Dutch processing and is therefore our product of choice.

On day 2 you will also see capers appear. If you're not so familiar with these, capers are those salty, dark-green, pellet-like things, and they have to be one of the most under-stated foods out there. Intriguingly, they're actually pickled flower buds, which grow in the Mediterranean before being handpicked. And boy, they hit the jackpot as a Sirtfood, being absolutely crammed full of the sirtuin-activating nutrients kaempferol and quercetin. Flavour-wise it's a case of big things coming in small packages as they sure do pack a punch. But, if you're not au fait with using them, don't feel intimidated. We'll soon have you falling head over heels for these diminutive nutrient superstars, which when combined with the right ingredients provide a beautifully distinctive and inimitable flavour to round off a dish in style.

On day 2, you will consume:

- 3 x Sirtfood green juice (pages 93–5)
- 1 x main meal (either standard or vegan option, see below)

Take the juices at separate times of the day (e.g. first thing in the morning, mid-morning and mid-afternoon) and select one of the standard or vegan meal options:

Turkey escalope with sage, capers and parsley
and spiced cauliflower 'couscous' (pages 176–7)

+

15–20g dark chocolate (85 per cent cocoa solids)

or

Kale and red onion dhal with buckwheat (vegan, pages 178–9)

+

15–20g dark chocolate (85 per cent cocoa solids)

DAY 3

You're now on to your third day, and while the format stays the same as days 1 and 2, it's time to spice things up a bit.

For thousands of years the chilli has been an integral part of gastronomic experience around the world. Since it was first brought back to Europe from a Columbus voyage in the late fifteenth century it has been rapidly accepted as a staple in our own cooking. On one level, it is baffling that we would be so enamoured by it. Its pungent heat is designed as a plant defence mechanism to cause pain and dissuade predators from feasting on it, yet we relish it. There is something almost mystical about the food and our infatuation with it.

Incredibly one study showed that eating chillies together even increases cooperation between individuals[91]. And, from a health perspective we know that their seductive heat is fantastic for activating our sirtuins and boosting our metabolism. The chilli's culinary applications are endless, offering an easy Sirtfood boost. While we appreciate not everyone is a fan of hot or spicy food, hopefully we can entice you to consider adding chilli in small amounts, especially with the most recent research showing that those who eat hot spicy foods three or more times a week have a 14 per cent lower death rate compared to those who eat them less than once a week[92]. As Thai food expert chef David Thompson said in an interview with *Time* magazine:

'the point of chilies, is not just the heat but the way they enhance the flavours of other ingredients. Chilli is not meant to swamp or overpower but act as a counterpoint to something salty or sour or sweet, or to heighten the sensation of textures.' Bird's eye (sometimes sold as 'Thai chillies') is our chilli of choice as this has the best Sirtfood credentials.

Today is also the last day that you will consume three daily green juices – tomorrow you'll reduce this to two – which makes now a good time to go over some of the other beverages we recommend on the Sirtfood Diet. We know about the health benefits of green tea, and the inclusion of water won't shock anyone, but what about coffee as a Sirtfood? Over half of us will drink at least one cup of coffee every day, yet it's tinged with guilt as we're led to believe coffee is a vice and somehow an unhealthy habit. Nothing could be further from the truth, with research showing coffee to be a veritable treasure trove of fantastic plant compounds with health benefits. This explains why coffee drinkers are at significantly less risk of diabetes[93], as well as certain cancers[94] and neurodegenerative disease[95]. As for the ultimate irony, instead of being a toxin, coffee actually protects our livers and makes them healthier[96]! So while we appreciate coffee is not for everyone, and some people can be very sensitive to the effects of caffeine, if you do enjoy coffee, then it's happy days as far as we are concerned.

On day 3, you will consume:

- 3 x Sirtfood green juice (pages 93–5)
- 1 x main meal (either standard or vegan option, see below)

Take the juices at separate times of the day (e.g. first thing in the morning, mid-morning and mid-afternoon) and select one of the standard or vegan meal options:

Aromatic chicken breast with kale and red onions and a tomato and chilli salsa (pages 180–1)

+

15–20g dark chocolate (85 per cent cocoa solids)

or

Harissa baked tofu with cauliflower 'couscous' (vegan, pages 182–3)

+

15–20g dark chocolate (85 per cent cocoa solids)

DAY 4

Day 4 has arrived, the halfway point on your journey to a lighter and leaner you. The big change to the previous three days is that you will now drop one of the daily green juices and replace it with a second daily meal. For today, and each of the remaining days, that means two green juices and two delicious Sirtfood-rich meals.

The inclusion of Medjool dates in a list of foods that stimulates weight loss and promotes health may come as a surprise. Especially when we tell you that Medjool dates contain a staggering 66 per cent sugar. Sugar possesses no sirtuin-activating properties whatsoever; rather it has well-established links to obesity, heart disease and diabetes – quite the opposite of what we are looking to achieve. But processed and refined sugar is very different from sugar carried in a vehicle provided by nature that is balanced with sirtuin-activating polyphenols: the Medjool date. In complete contrast to normal sugar, Medjool dates, eaten in moderation, actually have no real noticeable blood-sugar raising effects[97]. On the contrary, eating them is linked to having less diabetes and heart disease. They have been a staple food around the world for centuries and in recent years there has been an explosion in scientific interest in dates, and they are emerging as a potential medicine for a number of diseases[98, 99]. In that knowledge you can be assured their delicious inclusion in today's Sirt muesli only enhances its healthful benefits. Herein lies the uniqueness and power of the Sirtfood Diet: it refutes the dogma and allows you to indulge in sweet things in moderation without feeling guilty.

We are also adding chicory to the menu today. Like onion, red is best, but the yellow variety is also a Sirtfood. The red variety can be a bit harder to find but yellow is a perfectly suitable alternative. If you're ever stuck on how to increase chicory in your diet, you can't lose by adding its leaves to a salad where its welcome, tart flavour adds the perfect crunch to a zesty extra virgin olive oil-based dressing. For some it's an acquired taste but in the words of food writer Hugh Fearnley-Whittingstall, 'once you're hooked, there'll be no turning back.'

On day 4, you will consume:

- 2 x Sirtfood green juice (pages 93–5)
- 2 x main meal (either standard or vegan option, see below)

Take the juices at separate times of the day (e.g. the first juice either first thing in the morning or mid-morning, the second juice mid-afternoon) and select your meals from either the standard or vegan options:

MEAL 1: Sirt muesli (page 184)
MEAL 2: Pan-fried salmon fillet with caramelised chicory, rocket and celery leaf salad
(pages 185–6)

or

MEAL 1: Sirt muesli (page 184)
MEAL 2: Tuscan bean stew (vegan, pages 187–8)

DAY 5

You're on the march to day 5 already, and this is where things start to get a bit fruity. Fruit has been increasingly vilified in recent years, getting a bad rap in the growing fervour against sugar. Fortunately for berry lovers, such a maligned reputation could not be more ill deserved. Strawberries have a very low sugar content – they contain just one teaspoon of sugar per 100g. Additionally, strawberries have pronounced effects on improving how the body handles sugary carbohydrates. What researchers have found is that if we add strawberries to sugary carbohydrates it has the effect of reducing insulin demand, in essence turning the food into a sustained energy releaser[100]. So you can see strawberries are a fantastic inclusion in any weight loss and healthy diet. Strawberries are also delicious and extremely versatile as you will discover in this Sirtfood adaptation of the fresh and light Middle-Eastern classic tabbouleh.

Miso, meaning fermented beans, is a traditional Japanese food. Buddhist monks first discovered its amazing taste by grinding soy beans into a paste and fermenting them with salt and a naturally occurring fungus. Aside from its fantastic health-boosting properties, what miso really has to boast is its wonderful umami flavour, which ignites a savoury explosion on the taste buds. In our modern society we are more familiar with the notorious monosodium glutamate (MSG), which was artificially created to produce the same flavours. It goes without saying that deriving that magical umami taste from a traditional, natural and health-giving food is the way to go. Found as a paste in all good supermarkets and health-food shops, this should be a staple in all kitchens for adding an intense hit of flavour to dishes. As umami flavours enhance each other, miso goes extremely well with other savoury/umami foods, especially cooked protein, as you will taste yourself in today's tantalisingly tasty, quick and easy dishes.

On day 5, you will consume:

- 2 x Sirtfood green juice (pages 93–5)
- 2 x main meal (either standard or vegan option, see below)

Take the juices at separate times of the day (e.g. the first juice either first thing in the morning or mid-morning, the second juice mid-afternoon) and select your meals from either the standard or vegan options:

MEAL 1: Strawberry buckwheat tabbouleh (page 189)
MEAL 2: Miso marinated baked cod with stir-fried greens and sesame (pages 190–1)

or

MEAL 1: Strawberry buckwheat tabbouleh
(vegan, page 189)
MEAL 2: Soba (buckwheat noodles) in a miso broth with
tofu, celery and kale (vegan, pages 192–3)

DAY 6

According to ancient Greek historian Thucydides, 'the peoples of the Mediterranean began to emerge from barbarism when they learnt to cultivate the olive and the vine'. And there could not be two more quintessential Sirtfoods than olive oil and red wine.

Olive oil is the most renowned food of the traditional Mediterranean diet. The olive tree, also known as the 'immortal tree', is among the oldest-known cultivated trees in the world. And its oil has been revered ever since people started to squeeze olives in stone mortars to collect the oil, almost 7,000 years ago. Cited by Hippocrates as a 'cure all', a couple of millennia later modern science only affirms its wonderful health benefits. When it comes to olive oil, the key is to buy extra virgin. Virgin olive oil is obtained from the fruit solely by mechanical means under conditions that do not lead to the deterioration of the oil so you can be assured of the quality and polyphenol content. 'Extra virgin' refers to the first pressing of the fruit ('virgin' is the second pressing) so has the greatest taste and quality, and this is the one we strongly recommend you use.

And no Sirtfood menu would be complete without the inclusion of red wine, the original Sirtfood. Its content of the sirtuin activator resveratrol, along with other key sirtuin activators such as piceatannol, are what are believed to be a key reason for the long lives and slim figures associated with the traditional French way of life, and what sparked the whole Sirtfood frenzy. Of course wine does contain alcohol so consumption should be limited. But the good news is that resveratrol is quite heat stable, which makes cooking with it a perfect way to get it into the diet. While we are not proclaiming ourselves to be wine connoisseurs, we can tell you that Pinot Noir is our number one grape choice by virtue of the fact that it tops the league table for resveratrol content compared with other wines.

On day 6, you will consume:

- 2 x Sirtfood green juice (pages 93–5)
- 2 x main meal (either standard or vegan option, see below)

Take the juices at separate times of the day (e.g. the first juice either first thing in the morning or mid-morning, the second juice mid-afternoon) and select your meals from either the standard or vegan options:

MEAL 1: Sirt super salad (pages 194–5)
MEAL 2: Chargrilled beef with a red wine jus, onion rings, garlic kale and herb roasted potatoes (pages 196–9)

or

MEAL 1: Lentil Sirt super salad (vegan, pages 194–5)
MEAL 2: Kidney bean mole with baked potato (vegan, pages 200–1)

DAY 7

Day 7 marks your last day of the first phase of the Sirtfood Diet. But rather than the end, this is only the beginning, as you embark on a lifestyle change where Sirtfoods take centre stage on your plate. Today's menu is a perfect illustration of just how easy it is to integrate an abundance of Sirtfoods into your normal way of eating. It's about showing you that there need be nothing more to it than taking a culinary favourite, and with just a little bit of creativity, turning it into a Sirtfood feast.

Walnuts are such a great Sirtfood because they fly in the face of conventional thinking. High fat, high calorie, yet well established for reducing weight and metabolic disease. That's the power of sirtuin activation. Walnuts are also wonderfully versatile, great for use in baking, salads and simply as a snack.

Pesto is fast becoming a kitchen staple, being big on flavour, as well as an incredibly quick way to breathe life into even the simplest of dishes. Traditionally made with basil and pine nuts, with some simple switches you can make a super-easy parsley and walnut pesto. The result is a delicious dish now with the Sirtfood credentials to match the flavour.

We can also apply the same logic to an everyday meal like omelette. A family favourite, and as easy to give it its Sirtfood stripes as it is to prepare. We also include bacon in this omelette. Why? Simply because bacon goes great in this omelette. The Sirtfood Diet is about what we include not what we exclude, and one that fits in with a sustainable way of eating. After all, isn't that the real secret to achieving long-term weight loss and health?

On day 7, you will consume:

- 2 x Sirtfood green juice (pages 93–5)
- 2 x main meal (either standard or vegan option, see below)

Take the juices at separate times of the day (e.g. the first juice either first thing in the morning or mid-morning, the second juice mid-afternoon) and select your meals from either the standard or vegan options:

MEAL 1: Sirtfood omelette (pages 202–3)
MEAL 2: Baked chicken breast with walnut and parsley pesto and red onion salad (pages 204–5)

or

MEAL 1: Waldorf salad (vegan, page 206)
MEAL 2: Roasted aubergine wedges with walnut and parsley pesto and tomato salad (vegan, pages 207–8)

9

Phase 2: Maintenance

Congratulations on completing Phase 1 of the Sirtfood Diet! Already you should be seeing great results with fat loss and are not only looking slimmer and more toned, but feeling revitalised and re-energised. So, what now?

Having seen these often remarkable transformations ourselves first hand, we know how much you'll want not just to preserve all those benefits, but see even better results. After all, Sirtfoods are designed to be eaten for life. The question is how you adapt what you have been doing in Phase 1 into your usual dietary routine. That's exactly what prompted us to create a follow-on 14-day maintenance plan designed to help you make the transition from Phase 1 to your more normal dietary routine and thus help sustain and further extend the benefits of the Sirtfood Diet.

What to expect

During Phase 2, you will consolidate your weight loss results and continue to steadily lose weight.

Remember that the one striking thing we have found with the Sirtfood Diet is that most or all of the weight that people lose is from fat, and that many actually put on some muscle. So we want to remind you again not to judge your progress purely by the numbers on the scale. Look in the mirror to see if you are looking leaner and more toned, see how your clothes are fitting, and lap up the compliments that you will receive from others.

Remember too, that just as the weight loss will continue, so the health benefits will grow. By following the 14-day maintenance plan, you're really starting to lay down the foundations for a future of lifelong health.

How to follow Phase 2

The key to success in this phase is to keep packing your diet full of Sirtfoods. To make it as easy as possible, we've put together a seven-day menu plan for you to follow, including delicious family-friendly recipes, with each day packed to the rafters with Sirtfoods (though see page 162 for advice regarding children). All you need to do is repeat the seven-day plan twice to complete the 14 days of Phase 2.

On each of the 14 days your diet will consist of:

- 3 x balanced Sirtfood-rich meals
- 1 x Sirtfood green juice
- 1–2 x optional Sirtfood bite snacks

Once again, there are no rigid rules for when you have to consume these. Be flexible and fit it around your day. A few simple rules of thumb to remember are:

- Have your green juice either first thing in the morning, at least 30 minutes before breakfast, or mid-morning.
- Try your best to eat your evening meal by 7pm.

Portion sizes

Our focus during Phase 2 is not on counting calories. Over the long term this is not a practical, or even successful approach for the average person. Instead we're focusing on sensible portions, really well-balanced meals, and most importantly, filling up on Sirtfoods so you can continue to benefit from their fat-burning and health-promoting effects.

We have also constructed the meals in the plan to make them satiating, which will help you to stay feeling fuller for longer. That, combined with the natural appetite-regulating effects of Sirtfoods, means that you won't spend the next 14 days feeling hungry, but instead pleasantly satisfied, well fed and extremely well nourished.

Just as in Phase 1, remember to listen to your body and be guided by your appetite. If you prepare meals according to our instructions and find you are comfortably full before you've finished a meal, then just stop! Rather than eating until you feel stuffed, why not give a thought to the exceptionally long-lived Okinawans who live by the saying '*Hara hachi bu*', which means to eat until you are 80 per cent full.

What to drink

You will continue to include one green juice daily throughout Phase 2. This is to keep you topped up with high levels of Sirtfoods.

Just as in Phase 1, you can consume other fluids freely throughout Phase 2. Our preferred drinks for you to include are plain water, your home-made flavoured water, coffee and green tea. Remember that green tea and coffee are both Sirtfoods, so there's absolutely no need to feel guilty about continuing to enjoy a brew. Again, if your predilection is for black or white tea, feel free to enjoy. The same applies to herbal teas. The good news is that you can enjoy the occasional glass of red wine during Phase 2. Red wine is a Sirtfood due to its content of the sirt-activating polyphenols resveratrol and piceatannol, making it by far the best choice of alcoholic beverage. But, with alcohol itself having adverse effects on our fat cells, moderation is still best, and throughout Phase 2 we recommend limiting your intake to one glass of red wine with a meal, on two or three days per week.

Returning to three meals

For the last week you consumed just one or two meals a day, which gave you lots of flexibility over when you ate your meals. As we now return to a more normal routine, and the time-proven staple of three meals a day, it's a good time to talk about breakfast.

Eating a good breakfast sets us up for the day, increasing our energy and concentration levels. In terms of our metabolism, eating earlier keeps our blood sugar and fat levels in check. That breakfast is a good thing is borne out by a number of studies that typically show that people who regularly eat breakfast are less likely to be overweight.

The reason for this is down to our internal body clocks (see page 83). Our body expects us to eat early in anticipation of when we are going be most active and needing fuel. With our body primed for energy intake early in the day, we are much more likely to burn up this food for energy, whereas later in the day it is more likely to be stored as fat. This is exactly what we see among night-shift workers, who have higher rates of obesity and metabolic disease, which is at least partly due to the effects of their late eating patterns[101, 102].

Yet on any given day as many as a third of us will skip breakfast. It's a classic symptom of our busy modern lives and is most prominent among young professionals who are rushing out the door to work. With hectic lifestyles the perception is that there simply isn't enough time to eat well. But as you will see, with the nifty breakfasts we have laid out for you here, nothing could be further from the truth. From the Sirtfood smoothie which can be drunk on the go, to the pre-made Sirt muesli, or a quick and easy Sirtfood scrambled eggs/tofu, finding those extra few minutes in the morning will reap dividends not only for your day but your longer-term weight and health.

With Sirtfoods also working as additional regulators of our body clocks, there is even more to be gained by getting an early-morning hit of them. This is achieved not just through eating a Sirtfood-rich breakfast, but especially through the inclusion of the green juice, which we recommend you have either first thing in the morning – at least 30 minutes before breakfast – or mid-morning. From our own clinical experience, we do get many reports of people

117

who drink their green juice first thing and do not feel hungry for a couple of hours afterwards. If this is the effect it has on you, it is perfectly fine to wait a couple of hours before having breakfast. Just don't skip it. Alternatively, you can kick off your day with a good breakfast then wait two–three hours before having the green juice. Be flexible and just go with whatever works for you.

Sirtfood bites

When it comes to snacking, you can take it or leave it. There has been so much debate about whether eating frequent, smaller meals is best for weight loss, or whether you should just stick to three balanced meals a day. The truth is, it doesn't really matter.

The way we have constructed the maintenance menu for you ensures you will eat three well-balanced Sirtfood-rich meals per day, and you may find you really don't need a snack. But perhaps you've been busy in the office, working out or dashing around with the kids, and need something to tide you over to the next meal. And if that 'little something' is going to give you a whammy of Sirtfood nutrients and taste delicious, then it's happy days. This is why we created our 'Sirtfood bites'. These clever little snacks are a genuine guilt-free treat made entirely from Sirtfoods: dates, walnuts, cocoa, extra virgin olive oil and turmeric.

For days you need them, we recommend eating one, or a maximum of two, per day.

'Sirtifying' your meals

We've seen that the only sustainable diets are ones of inclusion not exclusion. But true success goes beyond this – it must be compatible with modern-day living. Whether it be the convenience to meet the demands of our hectic lives or fitting in with our role as the bon vivant at dinner parties, the way we eat should be hassle-free. You should be able to enjoy your svelte figure and radiant glow, instead of worrying about kooky food demands and restrictions.

What's so fantastic about Sirtfoods is that they are really accessible, familiar and easy to include in your diet. In the next section you will experience just how easily they fit in with normal day-to-day living. Here, as you bridge the gap between Phase 1 and routine eating, you will be building foundations for a new improved way of lifelong eating.

The key principle is what we call 'Sirtifying' your meals. This is where we take familiar dishes, including many classic favourites, and with some clever swaps and simple Sirtfood inclusions we keep all the great taste but add a ton more goodness. Throughout Phase 2 you will see just how easily this is achieved.

Examples include our delicious Sirtfood smoothie for the perfect on-the-go breakfast in a time-starved world. And the simple switch from wheat to buckwheat for adding extra taste and zip to the much-loved comfort food that is pasta. Meanwhile iconic, beloved dishes such as chilli con carne and curry don't even need much change, with the traditional recipes offering Sirtfood bonanzas. And who said 'fast food' meant bad food? We combine the authentic vibrant flavours of a pizza and remove the guilt when you make it yourself. There's no need to say farewell to indulgence either, as proven by our pancakes smothered with berries and dark chocolate sauce. It's not even dessert, it's breakfast, and it's great for you. Simple changes: you continue to eat the foods you love while driving a healthy weight and well-being. And that is the dietary revolution that are Sirtfoods.

Cooking for more

To embrace this we are now entering a 'Sirtfoods for all' stage, where recipes begin to cater for more mouths than one. Whether it be for family or friends, the new dinner recipes as well as the Sirtfood-packed soup we introduce in this section are designed with cooking for four in mind. And for those still cooking for one or two, why not take advantage of cooking batch meals for freezing to have meals ready for next week?

14-day meal plan

As well as our standard plan, we also have a meat-free version, which is suitable for both vegetarians and vegans. Feel free to go with whichever one you prefer, or even mix and match.

Each day you will consume:

- 1 x Sirtfood green juice (see pages 93-5)
- 3 x main meal (either standard or vegan options, see below)
- 1–2 x optional Sirt bites (see pages 235-6)

Consume the juice either first thing in the morning, at least 30 minutes before breakfast, or mid-morning.

	Breakfast
Day 8 and 15	Sirtfood smoothie (page 209)
or	Sirtfood smoothie (page 209)
Day 9 and 16	Sirt muesli (page 184)
or	Sirt muesli (page 184)
Day 10 and 17	Yoghurt with mixed berries, chopped walnuts and dark chocolate (page 215)
or	Soya or coconut yoghurt with mixed berries, chopped walnuts and dark chocolate (page 215)
Day 11 and 18	Spiced scrambled eggs (page 219)
or	Mushroom and tofu scramble (page 222–3)
Day 12 and 19	Sirtfood smoothie (page 209)
or	Sirtfood Smoothie (page 209)
Day 13 and 20	Buckwheat pancakes with strawberries, dark chocolate sauce and crushed walnuts (pages 227–229)
or	Soya or coconut yoghurt with mixed berries, chopped walnuts and dark chocolate (page 215)
Day 14 and 21	Sirtfood omelette (pages 202–3)
or	Sirt muesli (page 184)

Lunch	Dinner
Chicken Sirt super salad (pages 194–5)	Asian king prawn stir-fry with buckwheat noodles (pages 172–3)
Waldorf salad (page 206)	Tuscan bean stew (pages 187–8)
Stuffed wholemeal pitta (pages 210–11)	Butternut squash and date tagine with buckwheat (pages 212–13)
Butter bean and miso dip with celery sticks and oatcakes (page 214)	Butternut squash and date tagine with buckwheat (pages 212–13)
Tuna Sirt super salad (pages 194–5)	Chicken and kale curry with Bombay potatoes (pages 216–18)
Stuffed wholemeal pitta (pages 210–11)	Kale and red onion dhal with buckwheat (pages 178–9)
Strawberry buckwheat tabbouleh (page 189)	Sirt chilli con carne (pages 220–1)
Strawberry buckwheat tabbouleh (page 189)	Kidney bean mole with baked potato (pages 200–1)
Waldorf salad (page 206)	Smoked salmon pasta with chilli and rocket (pages 224–5)
Buckwheat pasta salad (page 226)	Harissa baked tofu with cauliflower 'couscous' (pages 182–3)
Tofu and shiitake mushroom soup (page 230)	Sirtfood pizza (pages 231–4)
Tofu and shiitake mushroom soup (page 230)	Sirtfood pizza (pages 231–4)
Lentil Sirt super salad (pages 194–5)	Baked chicken breast with walnut and parsley pesto and red onion salad (pages 204–5)
Lentil Sirt super salad (pages 194–5)	Miso and sesame glazed tofu with ginger and chilli stir-fried greens (pages 174–5)

10

Sirtfoods for Life

Congratulations, you've now finished both phases of the Sirtfood Diet! Let's just take stock of what you've achieved. You've completed the hyper-success phase, experiencing in the region of 7lb (3.2kg) weight loss, which likely includes some desirable muscle gain. You've consolidated that weight loss and further improved your body composition throughout the 14-day maintenance phase. Most importantly, you've marked the beginning of your own personal health revolution. You have taken a stand against the tide of ill health that so often strikes as we get older. Increased energy, vitality and well-being is the future you have chosen for yourself.

By now you will also be familiar with our top 20 Sirtfoods (see page 56) and have gained an appreciation of just how powerful they are. Not only that, but you will have become quite apt at including and enjoying them in your diet. It is imperative that these foods remain a prominent feature in your daily eating routine, for the continued weight loss and well-being they bring. But still, they are only 20 foods and after all, variety is the spice of life. So what next?

In this chapter we give you the blueprint for lifelong health. It's about getting your body in perfect balance with a diet that is suitable and sustainable for all, and provides all the health-enhancing nutrients we need. It's about continuing to reap the weight-loss rewards of the Sirtfood Diet using the very best foods that nature has to offer.

Beyond the top 20 Sirtfoods

We've seen why Sirtfoods are so beneficial: certain plants have sophisticated stress-response systems that produce compounds which activate sirtuins; the same fat-burning and longevity system in the body that is activated by fasting and exercise. The greater the amount of these compounds that plants produce in response to stress, the greater the benefit we obtain from eating them. Our list of the top 20 Sirtfoods is made up of the foods that really stand out by virtue of being especially packed full of these compounds, and thus the foods that have the most exceptional ability to impact body composition and well-being. Yet the sirtuin-activating effects of foods is not an all or nothing principle. There are many other plants out there which produce moderate levels of sirtuin-activating nutrients, and we encourage you to really expand the variety and diversity of your diet by eating these liberally too. The Sirtfood Diet is all about inclusion and the greater the variety of foods with sirtuin-activating properties that can be incorporated into the diet, the better. Especially if that means including even more of your favourite foods to max up the pleasure and enjoyment you can reap from your meals.

Let's use the analogy of exercise. The top 20 Sirtfoods are the (much more pleasurable) equivalent of sweating it out in the gym, with Phase 1 being the 'boot camp'. In contrast, eating those other foods with more moderate levels of sirtuin-activating nutrients is like reaping the rewards of going out for a good walk. Compare that to the typical standard diet with a nourishment value comparable to lying on the couch watching TV all day. Sure, sweating it out in the gym is good, but you'll soon get fed up with that if that's all you do. That walk should be encouraged too, especially if it means you are not choosing to lie on the couch instead.

For example, we included strawberries in our top 20 Sirtfoods as they are the most notable source of the sirtuin activator fisetin. Yet if we look more broadly at berries as a food group we find that they have benefits for metabolic health as well as promoting healthy aging. Reviewing their nutritional composition we find that other berries such as blackberries, blackcurrants, blueberries and raspberries also have notable levels of sirtuin-activating nutrients.

The same applies to nuts. Despite their calorific content, so beneficial are nuts that they actually promote weight loss and help shift inches from the waist. This is in addition to slashing the risk of chronic disease. While walnuts are our champion nut, sirtuin-activating nutrients are also found in chestnuts, pecans, pistachios and even peanuts.

Then we switch our attention to grains. There has been a growing aversion to grains in recent years in some quarters. Yet studies link wholegrain consumption to reduced inflammation, diabetes, heart disease and cancer. While they don't rival the Sirtfood credentials of the pseudo-grain buckwheat, we do see the presence of significant sirtuin-activating nutrients in other whole grains. And needless to say, when whole grains are processed into refined 'white' versions, their sirtuin-activating nutrient content is decimated. These refined versions are quite the toxic bunch, and are implicated in a plethora of modern-day health afflictions. We're not saying that you can never eat them, rather that you will be much better off sticking with the wholegrain version whenever you can.

For those who want to remain gluten-free, quinoa is a good Sirtfood source. And for a great wholegrain Sirtfood snack loved by all, look no further than popcorn.

Even infamous 'superfoods' get in on the act with the likes of goji berries and chia seeds having Sirtfood properties. This is most probably the unwitting reason for their observed health benefits. While it means they are indeed good for us to eat, we also know there are cheaper, more accessible and better options out there, so don't feel compelled to jump on that particular bandwagon. We see this same pattern across many food groups. Unsurprisingly, these are usually the ones that science has established are good for us and that we should be eating more of. Below we have listed an additional 40 foods which we have discovered also have Sirtfood properties. To maintain and continue your weight loss and well-being we actively encourage you to include these foods as you really expand the repertoire of your diet.

Vegetables
- artichokes
- asparagus
- bok choy/pak choi
- broccoli
- endive
- green beans
- shallots
- watercress
- white onions
- yellow chicory

Fruits
- apples
- black plums
- blackberries

- blackcurrants
- cranberries
- goji berries
- kumquats
- raspberries
- red grapes

Nuts and seeds
- chestnuts
- chia seeds
- peanuts
- pecan nuts
- pistachio nuts
- sunflower seeds

Grains and pseudo-grains
- popcorn
- quinoa
- wholemeal flour

Beans
- broad beans
- white beans (e.g. cannellini or haricot)

Herbs and spices
- chives
- dill (fresh and dried)

- dried oregano
- dried sage
- ginger
- peppermint (fresh and dried)
- standard chillies/hot peppers
- thyme (fresh and dried)

Beverages
- black tea
- white tea

Protein power

A high-protein diet is one of the most popularised diets of recent years. The consumption of higher amounts of protein, when dieting, has been found to promote satiety, maintain metabolism and reduce loss of muscle mass. But it's when Sirtfoods are combined with protein that things get taken to a whole new level.

As you may recall, protein is an essential inclusion in a Sirtfood-based diet to reap maximum benefits. Protein is made up of amino acids, and it is a specific amino acid, leucine, which powerfully complements the actions of Sirtfoods, enhancing their effects. Primarily, it does this by changing our cellular environment so that the sirtuin-activating nutrients from our diet work much more effectively. This means we get the best outcome from a Sirtfood-rich meal that is combined with leucine-rich protein. The best dietary sources of leucine include red meat, poultry, fish, seafood, eggs and dairy.

ANIMAL-BASED PROTEIN

In recent years animal products have been implicated as a contributing cause of many Western diseases, especially cancer. If that truly is the case, eating them with Sirtfoods might not seem such a bright idea. In order to lay that to rest, here's our lowdown.

One of the big concerns about dairy, is that it's not just a simple food but a highly sophisticated signalling system for inducing rapid body growth in offspring. While this has a valued purpose in early life, in adult life it may not be so appropriate. Persistent and hyper-activation of the key growth signal that dairy activates in the body (called mTOR) is now associated with aging and the development of age-related disorders such as obesity, type 2 diabetes, cancer and neurodegenerative diseases[103]. Despite the intricacies of this signalling system being a relatively new area of research and so still very much an unknown and theoretical risk, it lends validation to why people would shy away from dairy products. However, there is one thing research points to: if we add Sirtfoods to a diet containing dairy, they inhibit the inappropriate effects of mTOR on our cells, rescinding this risk, making Sirtfoods a must-include with a dairy-based diet[104].

Overall, reviews of dairy and cancer are mixed[105–107]. When we stack up all the research, in the context of a Sirtfood-rich diet, moderate dairy consumption is perfectly fine and can offer many valuable nutrients to complement Sirtfoods.

As well as being a valuable protein source, dairy is an excellent source of vitamins and minerals, such as iodine, calcium and phosphorous. Our recommendation for adults is to consume up to three servings of dairy (but no more than 1 litre of milk, or equivalent) a day.

When it comes to meat and cancer risk, poultry is perfectly okay, but red and processed meat are much more suspect. While evidence implicating them in breast and prostate cancer is pretty thin on the ground, there is legitimate concern that red and processed meat consumption plays a role in bowel cancer[108]. Processed meat seems the worst culprit. While there is no need to strike it off the menu completely, it should be included in just small amounts instead of being a staple.

When it comes to red meat the good news is that research shows that cooking red meat with Sirtfoods rescinds its cancer risk. Whether it be creating a marinade with herbs, spices and extra virgin olive oil, cooking your beef with onions, adding in a nice cup of green tea or indulging in after-dinner dark chocolate. These all pack a Sirtfood punch, which actually help to neutralise red meat's harmful effects[109-112]. While we are all for having your steak and eating it, don't go overboard. Red meat intake is best kept below 500g per week (cooked weight), which is roughly the equivalent of 700–750g raw.

Poultry is an excellent source of protein, along with vitamins and minerals such as B vitamins, potassium and phosphorous. Our recommendation for adults is to eat it freely.

Red meat is also an excellent source of protein, along with vitamins and minerals such as iron, zinc and vitamin B12. Our recommendation for adults is to eat up to a maximum of three servings a week.

Egg consumption and cancer risk has not been studied as thoroughly as meat and dairy products have, but in this regard there seems little reason for concern. Instead, what eggs have been implicated in causing is heart disease. This is because eggs are a major source of dietary cholesterol. Thus we are told to limit egg consumption. Interestingly, other countries, including Nepal, Thailand and South

Africa recommend consuming eggs as regularly as every day for their nutritional benefits. So who is right? The evidence is convincing in siding with the latter. Daily egg consumption is not linked to any increased risk of coronary heart disease or stroke[113]. While specific genetic conditions may require reduced dietary cholesterol intake, for the general population this restriction is not relevant.

As well as being a valuable protein source, eggs are an excellent source of essential nutrients such as B vitamins, vitamin A and carotenoids. Our recommendation for adults is to eat as desired as part of a balanced diet.

The power of three

The second major nutrient group that powerfully complements Sirtfoods are the omega-3 long chain fatty acids EPA and DHA. For years omega-3 has been the cherished favourite of the nutritional health world. What we didn't know previously, which we do now, is that they also enhance the activity of a subset of sirtuin genes in the body that are directly linked to longevity. This makes them the perfect pairing with Sirtfoods.

Omega-3s have potent effects in reducing inflammation and reducing the level of fats in the blood. To that we can add additional heart-healthy effects: they make the blood less likely to clot, stabilise the electrical rhythm of the heart and bring down blood pressure. Even the pharmaceutical industry is now turning to them as an aid in the battle against heart disease. And the litany of benefits doesn't end there. Omega-3s also affect the way we think, having been shown to improve mood as well as helping to stave off dementia.

When we talk about omega-3s we're essentially talking about eating fish, specifically the oily varieties, because no other dietary source comes close to providing the significant levels of EPA and DHA we need. And all we need to see the benefits is two servings of fish a week, with an emphasis on oily fish. Unfortunately we are not a big nation of fish eaters and less than a fifth of us achieve this. As a result our intake of the precious EPA and DHA comes up woefully short.

Plant foods such as nuts, seeds and green leafy vegetables also contain omega-3 but in a form called alpha-linolenic acid, which needs to be converted to EPA or DHA in the body. This conversion process is poor which means that alpha-linolenic acid provides a negligible amount of our omega-3 needs. Even with the wonderful benefits from Sirtfoods we should not overlook the added value that consuming sufficient levels of omega-3 fats brings. The best omega-3 fish sources are herring, sardines, salmon, trout and mackerel in that order. While fresh tuna is naturally high too, the majority of the omega-3 is lost in the tinned version. And for vegetarians and vegans, while plant sources should still be incorporated into the diet, a supplement of DHA-enriched microalgae (up to 300mg a day) is also encouraged.

> As well as being a valuable omega-3 and protein source, oily fish is an excellent source of vitamins and minerals such as vitamin A, B vitamins and trace minerals such as iodine and zinc. The recommendation for adults is to eat at least two servings of fish, of which one is oily fish, a week.

Can a Sirtfood Diet provide it all?

So far our focus has been solely on Sirtfoods and reaping their maximum benefits so that we can achieve the body we want and powerfully boost our health in the process. But is this a responsible dietary approach to be taking in the long term? After all there is more to diet than just sirtuin-activating nutrients. What about all the vitamins, minerals and fibre that are also essential for our well-being, and the foods we should be eating to satisfy those demands?

Intriguingly, what we find is that when we keep a strong focus on Sirtfoods, complemented by protein-rich foods and sources of omega-3, dietary needs are satisfied across the whole spectrum of essential nutrients. Much more so than any other diet in fact. For example, we include kale because it is a potent Sirtfood, yet, it is also a great source of vitamins C, K and folate, and the minerals manganese, calcium and magnesium. As well as immune-boosting beta-carotene, kale is also a tremendous source of the carotenoids lutein and zeaxanthin, both of which are critical in eye health.

Likewise, walnuts are rich in minerals including magnesium, copper, zinc, manganese, calcium and iron, as well as fibre. Buckwheat is full of manganese, copper, magnesium, potassium and fibre. Onions tick the boxes for vitamin B6, folate, potassium and fibre. And strawberries are excellent sources of vitamin C as well as potassium and manganese. And so it goes on.

Once you broaden your diet to include the extended Sirtfood list, as well as keeping room for all those other good foods you enjoy eating, unwittingly, what you will actually end up with is a diet far richer in vitamins, minerals and fibre than you ever had before. In effect, what Sirtfoods offer is a missing food group that changes the landscape of how we judge how good foods are for us, and how we eat a truly complete diet.

In fact, following a Sirtfood-based diet leaves a potential shortfall of only two key nutrients: selenium and vitamin D. This is not unexpected, however, as every diet runs the risk of missing these two nutrients simply because they occur in very low levels in our food supply. These are the two nutrients you should consider supplementing while following the Sirtfood Diet so let's give you the lowdown on each of them.

SELENIUM

Selenium is an impressive nutrient with key roles in supporting our immune system and keeping inflammation under control, with benefits also noted in fertility and thyroid function. Resistance to cancer, especially of the prostate, is its standout claim. Prostate cancer incidence was slashed in half when those who were deficient were supplemented[112]. Selenium enters our food supply through the soil, but sadly British and most other European soils are deficient. While the USA fares just fine, daily intakes in the UK are less than half of those needed, putting health at risk as a result.

As selenium now only enters our food supply in minute amounts, supplementation is warranted. Optimal levels, similar to those seen in the USA, are achieved through a dose of 50mcg a day for women and 100mcg a day for men.

Brazil nuts are often touted as an exceptional source of

selenium. Don't buy into that notion. While we would love there to be a food that could solve the selenium problem, unfortunately Brazil nuts contain undesirably high levels of barium, a toxic metal, and radium, a radioactive material[115]. Also, the selenium content of Brazil nuts is highly variable (as much as 1000-fold difference)[116], which is important because studies show consuming too much selenium is as bad for you as getting too little.

In the UK, and most of Europe, adult females should supplement their diet with 50mcg of selenium a day and adult males 100mcg a day. The best way to supplement this is in the form of selenium yeast. In the USA there is ample selenium in the food supply and no need to supplement.

VITAMIN D

Vitamin D has been the red-hot vitamin of the last decade. Known to be essential for bone health, there has been an explosion of research showing that vitamin D is also crucial for protection against cancer, heart disease, diabetes and autoimmune disease. But as the sunshine vitamin (we make it when the sun shines on our skin), dietary sources of vitamin D are severely limited. Even if you eat the richest dietary sources such as oily fish, eggs, liver, meat and fortified food, you're still going to fall way short of your needs. Diet typically provides less than 10 per cent of our vitamin D requirements, with more than 90 per cent coming from exposure to sunshine. Alas, in the UK we don't get too much sun. Even when we do, we're advised to slap on the sunblock which blocks vitamin D production by up to 98 per cent. So what do we do?

In the summer months we advise safe sun exposure. For example, as little as 4 minutes of summer sun exposure (without sunblock) to one quarter of your body (arms and legs) will give you your daily vitamin D quota. As set out in the 2010 unified view by the British Association of Dermatologists, Cancer Research UK, Diabetes UK, the Multiple Sclerosis Society, the National Heart Forum, the National Osteoporosis Society and the Primary Care Dermatology Society, total avoidance of the sun is not the aim. On the contrary, it's fine to go out in the sun in the middle of the day without sunscreen for just a few minutes, and this is all the time you need to make appreciable amounts of vitamin D.

In the winter months it's a different story. In the UK we cannot make vitamin D from the sun between the end of October and the end of March. This is when supplementation is required. A daily dose of 1,000IU will maintain desirable levels throughout this period.

For adults in all countries at latitude 41° and above (UK, Northern Europe and some of North America), safe sun during the summer and a daily supplement of 1,000IU between October and March will provide your vitamin D needs.

TOPPING UP PLANT-BASED DIETS

Sirtfoods are a celebration of the best plant foods on the planet. So it should come as no surprise that vegetarians, who naturally include more of them in their diet, have been shown to have lower rates of cancer, diabetes, heart disease and obesity. Authorities such as the prestigious American Dietetic Association are vociferous in their support of vegetarian diets, stating they are healthful, nutritionally adequate, and may provide health benefits in the prevention and treatment of certain diseases[117]. Plant-based cooking is worthy of its own plaudits and deserving of a place on anyone's dinner table. Already you will have experienced this for yourself, with the inclusion of dishes such as the Butternut squash and date tagine (see pages 212–13) in Phase 2 for both vegetarians and carnivores alike, offering plant-based fare at its best.

However, when it comes to eating solely plant-based vegan diets, it's a different matter. As good as Sirtfoods are, the diet can come up short. Without animal protein to complement Sirtfoods there is a risk of additional nutritional deficiency beyond selenium and vitamin D (see pages 138–41).

We've already seen how essential omega-3 fatty acids are for health and how plant sources are lacking. Thus our recommendation for vegetarians and vegans is for a DHA-enriched microalgae supplement to be taken daily.

Vegetarians and especially vegans can also find themselves lacking vitamin B12. We can only get vitamin B12 from animal products (including dairy and eggs), so eat nothing but plant foods and sooner or later you'll wind up deficient. If we become deficient in vitamin B12 we put ourselves at increased risk of heart disease, anaemia, neurological degeneration, depression and dementia. If you wish to eat a strictly plant-based diet, the best way around this conundrum is to take vitamin B12 in the form of a supplement.

Calcium is another key nutrient vegans need to be aware of: there is a 30 per cent greater incidence of fractures in vegans due to low calcium intake[118]. While it is possible to get calcium from a plant-based diet, you need to make a conscious effort. Good plant sources of calcium include green vegetables (e.g. kale, broccoli, bok choy), calcium-fortified beverages (soya milk, almond milk, rice milk), tofu set with calcium, nuts and seeds. Even still, a moderate calcium supplement may be required.

Finally, very high rates of iodine deficiency (80 per cent in vegans and 25 per cent in vegetarians)[119] have been found in people eating plant-based diets. While iodised salt is a very effective means of topping your iodine levels up, it is quite difficult to get in the UK. With dietary sources coming from fish, seafood and milk, vegans run into trouble. Iodine is vital for making thyroid hormones, which are absolutely critical in regulating metabolism, so unless vegans are using an appreciable amount of iodised salt, a supplement is probably required. While seaweed is a very rich source of iodine it can contain extremely high and potentially excessive levels, which is just as bad for the thyroid as getting too little, so should not be relied upon.

The physical activity effect

The Sirtfood Diet is about eating those foods designed by nature to promote sustained weight loss and well-being. But with the benefits you see from following it, it is possible to fall into the trap of thinking that there is no need to exercise. Many diet books will endorse this, saying how ineffective exercise is compared to following the correct diet for weight loss. And it's true, we cannot out-exercise a bad diet. As we saw earlier, it's not the way that was intended to drive weight loss. It's inefficient, and too much borders on being harmful. So, it's true that there's no need to pound the treadmill until we are seeing stars, or perform the feats of an Olympian, but what about general everyday movement?

The fact is we are far less active now than we used to be. The age of technology, for all the advances it has brought, has meant physical activity is virtually factored out of our daily lives. Unless we actually want to, we really don't have to bother with the whole business of being active. We can roll out of bed, drive to work, take the elevator, sit at a desk all day, drive home, eat, watch TV before rolling into bed again, then doing the same the next day, and the next.

Forget about weight loss for a moment and just take a look at the litany of health benefits being active is linked to. These include reduced risk of cardiovascular disease, stroke, hypertension, type 2 diabetes, osteoporosis, obesity and cancer as well as improved mood, sleep, confidence and sense of well-being. While a lot of the benefits of being active are driven through switching on our sirtuin genes we should not use eating Sirtfoods as a reason not to engage in exercise. Rather we should appreciate how being active is the perfect complement to our consumption of Sirtfoods. This stimulates maximum sirtuin activation, and all the benefits that brings, exactly as nature intended.

What we are talking about here is meeting government guidelines of 30 minutes of moderate physical activity five times a week. Moderate activity is the equivalent of a brisk walk. But it does not have to be restricted to this. Any sport or physical activity you enjoy is suitable. Enjoyment and exercise don't need to be mutually exclusive! And team or community sports are enriched all the more by their social aspect. It's about day-to-day things too, like taking the bike instead of the car. Or getting off the bus a stop earlier, or simply parking further away to increase the distance you have to walk. Take the stairs instead of the elevator. Go outside and do some gardening. Play with your kids in the park, or get out more with the dog. It all counts. Performed regularly, and at moderate intensity, anything that has you up and moving will activate your sirtuin genes, enhancing the benefits of the Sirtfood Diet.

Engaging in physical activity while eating a Sirtfood-rich diet gives maximum sirtuin bang for your buck. All that is needed to achieve the physical activity effect is the equivalent of a brisk 30-minute walk five times a week.

SUMMARY

- While the top 20 Sirtfoods should remain centre plate, there are many other plants with sirtuin-activating properties that should be included in our diets to make them varied and diverse.

The Sirtfood Diet

- A diet rich in Sirtfoods complemented by the inclusion of animal products and fish provides all the benefits of sirtuin activation, as well as meeting the need for other essential nutrients.

- Like any diet, a Sirtfood Diet will be unable to meet our selenium and vitamin D needs so it is important to consider supplementing.

- While vegans and vegetarians can get all the benefits from a Sirtfood-based diet, careful attention should be given to those nutrients that may be lacking and appropriate food choices or supplementation made.

- Followers of the Sirtfood Diet are encouraged to engage in moderate activity for 30 minutes five times a week to reap the many benefits of exercise for well-being and stimulate maximum sirtuin activation.

11

Sirtfoods for All

As we journeyed deeper and deeper into the wonderful world of Sirtfoods, we began to realise just how wide their application could be. We're very aware that no two people eat the same, and many health-conscious people are strongly committed to a certain way of eating, with the likes of intermittent fasting, low-carb, paleo and gluten-free diets being especially popular. While they don't work for some, others swear by them. But just how do Sirtfoods fit in with these?

A light-bulb moment struck with the realisation that every single one of these popular diets would be greatly enhanced if Sirtfoods were integrated into them. The benefits people were deriving from them – health or weight loss – could be amplified simply through the addition of Sirtfoods in sufficient quantities. In this way, Sirtfoods are universal: if there's a way of eating that really works for you, incorporating Sirtfoods into it will make your results even better.

We're both busy clinicians and as our enthusiasm for Sirtfoods has grown, we have integrated Sirtfoods more and more strongly into the diets of the clients we work with, no matter what their preferred way of eating. Our conclusion is clear: not only are Sirtfoods compatible with all other dietary approaches, they powerfully enhance them. In fact, they should be essential ingredients in every popular diet. Overlook them and you're really missing a trick.

Intermittent fasting / 5:2 Diet

Intermittent fasting, also known as IF, has become a huge dietary phenomenon in the last few years, epitomised by the runaway success of the 5:2 Diet. This typically involves restricting calorie intake to 500–600 calories per day on two days per week, and eating whatever you want on the other five days.

While solid research into the benefits of intermittent fasting is still pretty limited, it does appear to be beneficial for weight loss and improving some of the risk factors for disease. But as we've seen; it's not suitable for large groups of the population, it causes undesirable muscle loss and it's only effective if you can stick to it. And that really is the elephant in the room when it comes to intermittent fasting and why we're not overly enamoured with it. In our clinical experience, the majority of people fail to stick to intermittent fasting regimes for any appreciable length of time. Hunger is an unpleasant feeling that gnaws away at you, so unsurprisingly people just don't like to feel hungry that often.

While intermittent fasting has not turned out to be a panacea, it is popular for a reason and there will be its fans who swear by its benefits. We fully respect this, of course. But why not give your fast a serious upgrade by 'Sirtifying' it?

With the introduction of Sirtfoods you will get all the benefits they bring to reduce the adverse effects of fasting, including helping to satiate hunger and preserve muscle. But there's another big bonus to their inclusion. You will remember that the benefits of fasting are mediated through the activation of our sirtuin genes, which is also exactly how Sirtfoods work. This means with Sirtfoods now present to share the fasting 'burden' you can up your calorie intake to a much more manageable level while still reaping all the same benefits.

This is exactly what we have found in our clinical practice. With just the inclusion of Sirtfood-rich green juices (the one used in this book) to a normal IF menu, followers have been able to increase their energy intake from a severe 500–600 calories on fast days to a much more manageable 800–1,000 calories.

So if your penchant is for intermittent fasting, you're missing a trick and making fast days unduly gruelling by not embracing Sirtfoods. In fact, there's a whole other angle where intermittent fasting diets would benefit by embracing Sirtfoods. With intermittent fasting diets there's very little, if any, focus on the *quality* of the diet; it's all about the calorie deficit on fast days. In fact, proponents are vociferous in endorsing the idea that you can eat whatever you want on non-fast days. Whether what you eat is good, bad or outright terrible, it seems it doesn't really matter. But, as we know, the body needs a continuous supply of essential nutrients to keep everything working in tip-top shape. Can we really expect to get away with depriving the body of critical nutrition, by eating whatever nutrient-stripped, processed foods we want, even if we are fasting for two days, and stave off chronic diseases like Alzheimer's or heart disease?

What if, on the other hand, you also included nutrient-dense Sirtfoods on your non-fasting days? You would no longer be burning fat and enhancing health two days a week, it would now be seven. To us this evolution of the intermittent fasting approach is a no-brainer. It's the equivalent of upgrading a black and white TV to HD.

Low-carb diet

Ever since Atkins, the father of low-carb diets, rose to meteoric notoriety, low-carb diets have been a major landmark on the weight-loss map. Subsequent reincarnations, such as the Dukan Diet, have continued to fuel the low-carb movement. Between them, they have notched diet-book sales up to the tens of millions. While such low-carb diets can be extreme, especially in their early 'assault' phases, their broad sentiments do reflect a wider shift in opinion toward an anti-sugar and even anti-carb stance. Increasingly people are abandoning the sinking ship of the low-fat paradigm and shifting allegiances to the 'carbs are the enemy' camp.

One of the beauties of the Sirtfood Diet is that it doesn't involve this territorial conflict. It's a diet of inclusion, which means that you really don't have to choose sides and exclude a whole food group from your diet in order to achieve the body you want. Nevertheless, we appreciate that many people have a preference for a lower-carb style of eating, so where do Sirtfoods fit in?

If your persuasion is toward low carb, then we urge you not to scrimp on Sirtfoods, but to embrace them. In our clinical experience, one of the biggest traps we see people fall into when eating low-carb-style diets is the lack of plant-based foods they contain. Meals become heavily oriented around meats (and often processed meats), fish, eggs, cheese and other dairy products, and plant-based foods get relegated in the pecking order. But if it's low carb, it's all good . . . Or so we're told.

Alas, the idea that plant-based foods aren't of central

importance in our diets flies in the face of virtually everything we know about diet and health. A diet depleted in the vast array of beneficial compounds found in plant foods will do little to avert an avalanche of chronic diseases such as dementia, heart disease and cancer. Yet it is perfectly possible to integrate an abundance of Sirtfoods into a carb-restricted way of eating. Just look at the top 20 list of Sirtfoods and you will discover that a vast majority of them are inherently low in carbs. We're talking about a bounty of leafy and low-carb vegetables (celery, chicory, kale, rocket, onions), culinary herbs (lovage, parsley), spices (bird's eye chilli, turmeric), capers, walnuts, cocoa, extra virgin olive oil, not forgetting the beverages (coffee and green tea). As for fruit, so often the target of attack on low-carb diets, even the strawberries weigh in with a mere teaspoon of carbohydrates from a generous 100g serving.

For us the bottom line is this: no low-carb diet should be a low-Sirtfood diet. Not only does incorporating Sirtfoods enhance the weight-loss benefits of a low-carb diet, but it dramatically increases its health potential.

Paleo diet

In a nutshell, the paleo diet promotes the idea that we should eat the foods that it is presumed our ancient ancestors were eating, before the advent of modern agriculture and more recently industrial food processing. In essence we're talking a hunter-gatherer- or caveman-style of diet, consisting of meats, fish and shellfish, vegetables, fruits and nuts, while exiled to the wilderness are dairy products, cereal grains, sugar and all processed foods.

For paleo dieters, we pose this question: what could be more paleo than eating the plant foods which we've co-evolved with that switch on our ancient sirtuin genes? You will recall that both plants and animals have developed ways of coping with common environmental stresses such as dehydration, sun exposure, lack of nutrients and attack by aggressors. Because of their sedentary nature (plants can't run away!), plants have developed especially sophisticated stress-response systems, producing a complex array of polyphenols that allow them to cope with their environment. For millennia, humans have been ingesting these polyphenols, piggybacking on these sophisticated stress-response signals produced by plants and reaping huge benefits as they switch on our own sirtuin genes.

What could be more paleo than consuming the sirtuin-activating plant compounds our hunter-gatherer forebears would have thrived on? Sirtfoods are the missing piece of the paleo philosophy.

Gluten-free diet

The beauty of the Sirtfood Diet for anyone who needs to avoid gluten is that the top 20 Sirtfoods are all naturally gluten-free. Gluten is a type of protein found in wheat, rye and barley. Some people with gluten intolerance can also be sensitive to oats (through cross-contamination). Sufferers of the autoimmune disease, coeliac disease, which affects about 1 in 100 people in the UK and Europe, are hyper-sensitive to gluten and cannot consume it in any form, but aside from this very serious gluten intolerance, many people are increasingly experimenting with gluten-free diets and often find they feel better on them.

When people embark on gluten-free diets, which involves cutting out staple foods like bread, pasta and the myriad of other foods made from gluten-containing grains, one of the big concerns is that the diet becomes nutritionally incomplete and no longer provides the full range of nutrients and fibre needed to stay in good health. What's so great about the Sirtfood Diet is that one of our top Sirtfoods is buckwheat, a naturally gluten-free and highly nutritious 'pseudo' grain, which as we have seen through the preceding chapters, is versatile enough to step in as a replacement for gluten-containing grains whether in the form of flour, pasta, flakes or noodles (check the packet carefully to ensure these are 100 per cent buckwheat).

Of course, the best diets are the ones that are diverse

and varied not repetitive and monotonous. We saw that quinoa, another 'pseudo' grain, is not only gluten-free, but also has noteworthy amounts of sirtuin-activating nutrients, making it the perfect back-up to buckwheat. Aside from eating it as a grain, quinoa is increasingly available in the form of flour, flakes and pasta from health-food stores and specialist online suppliers. With quinoa and buckwheat taking centre stage it's happy days for anyone adopting a gluten-free diet as not only do they offer a convenient alternative to other grains but including them as staple foods adds some serious Sirtfood credentials to the average diet.

We cannot leave the topic of gluten-free diets without a word of warning about the mass of gluten-free 'junk food' that now fills up the 'free from' shelves in every supermarket. These are the highly processed, refined, sugary, gluten-free alternatives to cakes, biscuits, cookies, breakfast cereals and so on. This has become a huge industry, but please don't fall into the trap of thinking that just because a product is 'gluten-free' that it is necessarily healthy. The majority of these foods are nutritionally empty junk, just like their gluten-containing counterparts. If you are following a gluten-free diet, we urge you to fill up on a diet rich in naturally gluten-free Sirtfoods, not gluten-free junk, and take your health and well-being to a whole new level.

SUMMARY

- Sirtfoods are not only compatible with all other dietary approaches but powerfully enhance their benefits.

- Eating a diet rich in Sirtfoods means that the calorie restriction of intermittent fasting can be less severe, yet the benefits will be the same if not greater.

- Low-carb diets that lack plant-based foods can be dramatically enhanced by the inclusion of Sirtfoods.

- Sirtfoods are the archetypal paleo foods, containing the sirtuin-activating polyphenols that humans would have evolved eating and reaping the benefits from over countless millennia.

- The top 20 Sirtfoods are naturally gluten-free making them a boon for anyone following a gluten-free diet.

12

Questions and Answers

SHOULD I EXERCISE DURING PHASE 1?

Regular exercise is one of the best things you can do for your health, and doing some moderate exercise will enhance the weight loss and health benefits of Phase 1 of the diet. As a general rule, we encourage you to continue your normal level of exercise and physical activity through the first seven days of the Sirtfood Diet. However, we suggest staying within your normal comfort zone as very prolonged or too-intense exercise may simply place too much stress on the body for this period. Listen to your body. There's no need to push yourself to do more exercise during Phase 1, let the Sirtfoods do the hard work instead.

I'M ALREADY SLIM – CAN I STILL FOLLOW THE DIET?

We do not recommend Phase 1 of the Sirtfood Diet for anyone who is underweight. A good way to find out if you are underweight is to calculate your Body Mass Index or BMI. As long as you know your height and weight, you can easily calculate this by using one of the numerous BMI calculators online. If your BMI is 18.5 or less, we don't recommend that you embark on Phase 1 of the diet. If your BMI is between 18.5 and 20, we would still urge caution as following the diet may mean that your BMI falls below 18.5. While many people aspire to be super-skinny, the reality is that being underweight can negatively affect many aspects of health, such as a lowered immune system, an elevated risk of osteoporosis (weakening of the bones), and fertility problems. While we don't recommend Phase 1 of the diet if you are underweight, we do still encourage the integration of plenty of Sirtfoods into a balanced way of eating so that all the health benefits of these foods can be reaped.

However, if you are slim, but have a BMI in the healthy range (20–25), there is absolutely nothing stopping you from getting started. A majority of the participants involved in the pilot trial had a BMI in the healthy range, yet still lost impressive amounts of weight and became more toned. Importantly, many participants reported a significant improvement in energy levels, vitality and appearance. Remember that the Sirtfood Diet is about promoting health as much as it is losing weight.

I'M OBESE – IS THE SIRTFOOD DIET RIGHT FOR ME?

Yes! Don't be put off by the fact that only a small minority of the participants who embarked on our pilot study were obese. This is because the pilot study was carried out in a health and fitness club where people are generally fitter and more health-conscious. Instead, be spurred on by the fact that the few who were obese had even better results than our healthy weight participants. Based on the research into sirtuin activation, you should also stand to reap the greatest changes in your well-being too. Being obese increases the risk of numerous chronic health problems, yet these are the very illnesses that Sirtfoods help to protect against.

I'VE REACHED MY TARGET WEIGHT AND DON'T WANT TO LOSE ANY MORE – DO I STOP EATING SIRTFOODS?

Firstly, congratulations on your weight-loss achievement! You've had great success with Sirtfoods but it does not end now. While we do not recommend further calorie restriction, your diet should still provide ample Sirtfoods. Many of our clients are now at their ideal body composition but continue to eat Sirtfood-rich diets. The great thing about

Sirtfoods is that they are a way for life. The best way to think about them with regards to weight management is that they help bring the body to the weight and composition it was meant to be. From here they work to maintain and keep you looking and feeling great. This is ultimately the goal we desire for all Sirtfood Diet followers.

I'VE FINISHED PHASE 2 – DO I STOP DRINKING THE MORNING SIRTFOOD GREEN JUICE NOW?

The green juice is our favourite way to get a fantastic hit of Sirtfoods to start your day, so we endorse its long-term consumption. Our Sirtfood green juice was carefully designed to include ingredients that provide a full spectrum of sirtuin-activating nutrients in potent fat-burning and well-being boosting doses. However, we are all for variety and while we do recommend you continue with a morning juice, we fully support anyone looking to experiment with different Sirtfood juice concoctions.

I TAKE MEDICATION – IS IT OKAY TO FOLLOW THE DIET?

The Sirtfood Diet is suitable for most people, but because of its powerful effects on fat burning and health it can alter certain disease processes and the actions of medication prescribed by your doctor. Likewise certain medications are not suitable in a fasted state.

During the trial of the Sirtfood Diet, we assessed the suitability of each person before they embarked on the diet, especially those who were taking medication. Obviously we can't do that for you, so if you suffer from a significant health problem, take prescribed medications, or have other reasons to be concerned about embarking on the diet, we recommend you discuss it with your doctor first. The chances are it will be fine and actually of profound benefit for you but it's important to check.

CAN I FOLLOW THE DIET IF I'M PREGNANT?

We don't recommend embarking on the Sirtfood Diet if you are trying to conceive or if you are pregnant or breast-feeding. It is a powerful weight-loss diet, which makes it unsuitable. However, don't be put off including plenty of Sirtfoods as these are exceptionally healthy foods to include as part of a balanced and varied diet for pregnancy. You will want to avoid red wine, due to its alcohol content, and limit caffeinated items such as coffee, green tea and cocoa as current UK government advice is not to exceed 200mg per day of caffeine in pregnancy (one mug of instant coffee typically contains 100mg of caffeine). Recommendations are not to exceed four cups of green tea daily and avoid matcha altogether. Other than that, you're free to reap the benefits of including Sirtfoods in your diet.

ARE SIRTFOODS SUITABLE FOR CHILDREN?

The Sirtfood Diet is a powerful weight-loss diet and not designed for children. However, that doesn't mean that children should miss out on including more Sirtfoods in their general diet for their excellent health benefits. A vast majority of Sirtfoods represent extremely healthy foods for children and help them achieve balanced and nutritious diets. Many of the recipes designed for Phase 2 of the diet were created with families in mind, including children's taste buds. The likes of the Sirtfood pizza (pages 231–4), the chilli con carne (pages 220–1) and the Sirtfood bites (pages 235–6) are perfect child-friendly foods with a superior nutritional value to usual food offerings for children.

While the majority of Sirtfoods are extremely healthy foods for children to eat, we do not recommend the green juice, which is too concentrated in fat-burning Sirtfoods. We also advise against significant sources of caffeine as would be found in coffee and green tea. You will also need to be careful with the inclusion of chillies and may opt to keep things milder for children.

WILL I GET A HEADACHE OR FEEL TIRED DURING PHASE 1?

Phase 1 of the Sirtfood Diet provides powerful naturally occurring food compounds in amounts that most people would not get in their normal diet and certain people can react as they adapt to this dramatic nutritional change. This can include symptoms such as a mild headache or tiredness, although these effects are in our experience mild and short-lived.

Of course, if symptoms are severe, or give you reason for concern, we recommend you seek prompt medical advice. Saying that, we have never seen anything other than occasional mild symptoms that resolve quickly, and within a few days most people find they have a renewed sense of energy, vigour and well-being.

SHOULD I TAKE SUPPLEMENTS?

Unless specifically prescribed for you by your doctor or other health-care professional, we do not recommend indiscriminate use of nutritional supplements. You will be ingesting a vast and synergistic array of natural-plant compounds from Sirtfoods, and it is these that will do you good. You cannot replicate these benefits with nutritional supplements and in fact, some nutritional supplements, especially if taken at high doses, may actually interfere with the beneficial effects of Sirtfoods, which is the last thing you want.

But are there any nutrients that fall short in our diet which may need topping up? Whenever possible, we think it is much better to get the nutrients you need from eating a balanced diet rich in Sirtfoods, than from taking nutrients in pill form. However, it is very difficult to get every single nutrient you need in optimum amounts, no matter how hard you try. The two nutrients you are likely to fall short of are vitamin D (through the winter months) and selenium. Our specific recommendations for those can be found on pages 138–41. Vegans will also have special nutritional considerations and our specific recommendations for those following purely plant-based diets can also be found on pages 141–3.

HOW OFTEN CAN I REPEAT PHASES 1 AND 2?

Phase 1 can be repeated again if you feel like you need a weight-loss or health boost, although we find most people do not need to repeat it any more frequently than at most once every three months. Instead, if you find you've gone off-track, need some fine-tuning or a bit more Sirtfood intensity, we recommend repeating some or all days of the Phase 2 section as often as you like. After all, Phase 2 is all about establishing a lifelong way of eating. Because the beauty of the Sirtfood Diet is that it doesn't require you to feel like you are endlessly on a 'diet', but instead is the springboard to developing lifelong positive dietary changes that create a lighter, leaner and healthier you.

I'VE READ ABOUT SUPERFOODS – SHOULD I BE INCLUDING THESE IN MY DIET TOO?

The first thing you need to know about the term 'superfood' is that it is not a scientific term at all but a marketing slogan. You do not need to concern yourself with so-called superfoods as the Sirtfood Diet brings together the healthiest foods on the planet into a revolutionary new way of eating. Just like it is a mistake to rely on taking a simple vitamin pill to make us healthy, so too it is a mistake to rely on a single so-called 'superfood' to do the same. It is the whole diet, made up of a whole spectrum of Sirtfoods and their vast array of natural compounds, acting in synergy, which is the true secret to achieving weight loss and lifelong health.

DO I HAVE TO DO PHASE 1 FOR SEVEN DAYS – CAN I DO FEWER?

There's nothing magical about Phase 1 being seven days. It is simply what we decided upon for our trial. We opted for that because it was long enough to get impressive results, but not so long that it became arduous. It also fits neatly into people's lives. Seven days is what was trialled and what is proven to be effective. However, if for whatever reason you find that you need to cut it short by a day or two, do so by completing up to the end of day 5 or day 6. Don't worry, you will still reap the lion's share of the benefits.

CAN I EAT WHATEVER I WANT ONCE I EAT PLENTY OF SIRTFOODS AND STILL SEE RESULTS?

One of the key reasons the Sirtfood Diet works so well long term is that it promotes good food instead of demonising bad food. Diets of exclusion simply do not work long term. It is true that processed foods that are high in sugars and fats reduce sirtuin activity in the body and thus a high consumption will reduce the benefits of Sirtfoods. However, if you keep your focus on consuming a diet rich in Sirtfoods, in our experience you will find that you are pleasantly satisfied and will have less desire for those processed foods and end up consuming far less junk than the average person as a result. If you do occasionally find yourself indulging in these processed foods, don't worry about it, as the power of Sirtfoods the rest of the time will make sure you still reap the benefits.

CAN I EAT AS MANY SIRTFOODS, EVEN THE HIGH-CALORIE ONES, AS I LIKE AND STILL LOSE WEIGHT?

Yes! Remember calories and calorie counting is a modern-day 'advancement'. Across the cultures and countless generations that have benefited from Sirtfoods such a concept did not exist, and there simply was no need. People ate as they felt like it, and stayed slim and free of disease.

Between their effects on regulating metabolism and appetite, you simply do not need to worry about eating too many Sirtfoods. While this is not an invitation to an all-you-can-eat challenge, feel free to eat as much Sirtfood as you like to satisfy your natural appetite. Our one exception is Medjool dates. Their inclusion showcases how high-sugar foods do not have to be bad for you when eaten in the form nature intended, and in moderation. But moderation is key here to making dates a guilt-free indulgent treat. In terms of drinks, when it comes to red wine consumption, it goes without saying it should be drunk responsibly and safely within government recommendations.

IS ORGANIC BETTER?

In an ideal world, we would encourage you to opt for organic produce where possible, practical and affordable. While there is little evidence that levels of conventional vitamins and minerals differ between organic and non-organic produce, what about the sirtuin-activating nutrients?

It is likely that organic produce carries a richer content of sirtuin-activating nutrients. Remember that the sirtuin-activating polyphenols found in plant foods are produced in response to environmental stresses, and without the intense use of pesticides, organically grown produce will have to battle that bit harder to deter and ward off environmental predators. This is likely to result in higher levels of polyphenols being produced, making organic produce potentially a more powerful Sirtfood than its non-organic equivalent. While organic is preferable, you will still get great results from the Sirtfood Diet if you opt for non-organic produce. Organic is just the cherry on top.

WHERE ARE THE BEST PLACES TO GET THE PRODUCTS USED IN THE DIET?

The Sirtfood Diet is a diet of inclusion, and the vast majority of the foods recommended are widely available and highly accessible, wherever you shop. A small handful of Sirtfoods and ingredients used in the recipes are less well known, and we appreciate you might need to be pointed in the right direction for those. Also, we've discovered a few useful tips along the way, such as which chocolate products are alkalised (which destroys many of the beneficial flavanols) and which are not, which we wanted to share with you.

Chocolate: Our go-to chocolate is Lindt Excellence 85% Cocoa. We were informed by Lindt that this is not alkalised (though their 90% is alkalised, so higher percentages are not necessarily better), therefore it retains higher levels of beneficial cocoa flavanols. Our cocoa powders of choice, for the same reason, are Rowntree's in the UK and Hershey's Natural in the USA.

Matcha: We like Do Matcha's offering (www.domatcha.co.uk) because it offers a much cheaper second-harvest product, compared with the expensive ceremonial-grade versions. This is perfect because not only is it more affordable but if anything the levels of sirtuin-activating nutrients are actually higher in the second-harvest product, most likely because of extended exposure to environmental stress.

Buckwheat: Buckwheat in its wholegrain form, and as a flour, is widely available in most supermarkets, but some of the buckwheat products we recommend in the recipes can be less easy to get hold of. Many of these will be available in good health-food shops or from other specialist online suppliers. Here are some other buckwheat sources we have found:

- Pasta (buckwheat spirals) from Orgran (www.orgran.com)
- Noodles (organic Japanese Soba 100 per cent buckwheat) from Clearspring (www.clearspring.co.uk)
- Flakes and puffs: www.bigoz.co.uk

13

Recipes

Some important notes about these recipes:

- Bird's eye chillies (sometimes sold as 'Thai chillies') are one of the top 20 Sirtfoods and appear regularly throughout these recipes. If you have never tried them, they are notably hotter than normal chillies. If you are not used to spicy food, we suggest starting off with half the chilli amount stated in the recipe, as well as deseeding your chilli before use. From here you can adjust the heat to your preference throughout the diet.
- Miso is a delicious flavour-packed fermented soya bean paste. You will find it comes in a range of colours, typically white, yellow, red and brown. The lighter-coloured miso pastes are sweeter than the dark ones, which can be quite salty. For our recipes brown

or red miso will work well, but by all means experiment and see which flavour you prefer. Red miso tends to be the saltier of these so if you do opt for this one, you might prefer to use a little less of it. The flavour and saltiness of miso can also vary between brands, so the best bet would be to check whatever type you buy and adjust the amount you use accordingly, so it's not too overpowering. That means a little trial and error, but you'll soon get the hang of it.

- If you haven't cooked buckwheat before, it couldn't be easier. We recommend that you first thoroughly wash the buckwheat in a sieve before placing in a pan of boiling water. Cooking times can vary so do check the instructions on your packet.

- Flat-leaf parsley would be best for all the dishes but if you can't get hold of it then curly will do.

- Onions, garlic and ginger are always peeled unless otherwise stated.

- Salt and pepper are not used in these recipes but feel free to season with sea salt and black pepper to your own taste preferences. Sirtfoods offer so much flavour you will likely find you do not need as much as you normally use.

Asian king prawn stir-fry with buckwheat noodles

SERVES 1

150g shelled raw king prawns, deveined
2 tsp tamari (you can use soy sauce if you are not avoiding gluten)
2 tsp extra virgin olive oil
75g soba (buckwheat noodles)
1 garlic clove, finely chopped
1 bird's eye chilli, finely chopped
1 tsp finely chopped fresh ginger
20g red onions, sliced
40g celery, trimmed and sliced
75g green beans, chopped
50g kale, roughly chopped
100ml chicken stock
5g lovage or celery leaves

Heat a frying pan over a high heat, then cook the prawns in 1 teaspoon of the tamari and 1 teaspoon of the oil for 2–3 minutes. Transfer the prawns to a plate. Wipe the pan out with kitchen paper, as you're going to use it again.

Cook the noodles in boiling water for 5–8 minutes or as directed on the packet. Drain and set aside.

Meanwhile, fry the garlic, chilli and ginger, red onion, celery, beans and kale in the remaining oil over a medium–high heat for 2–3 minutes. Add the stock and bring to the boil, then simmer for a minute or two, until the vegetables are cooked but still crunchy.

Add the prawns, noodles and lovage/celery leaves to the pan, bring back to the boil then remove from the heat and serve.

Miso and sesame glazed tofu with ginger and chilli stir-fried greens

SERVES 1

1 tbsp mirin

20g miso paste

1 x 150g block firm tofu

40g celery, trimmed

35g red onion

120g courgette

1 bird's eye chilli

1 garlic clove

1 tsp finely chopped fresh ginger

50g kale, chopped

2 tsp sesame seeds

35g buckwheat

1 tsp ground turmeric

2 tsp extra virgin olive oil

1 tsp tamari (soy sauce can be used if you are not avoiding gluten)

Heat the oven to 200°C/gas 6. Line a small roasting tin with greaseproof paper.

Mix the mirin and miso together. Cut the tofu lengthways, then cut each piece in half into triangles. Cover the tofu with the miso mixture and leave to marinate while you prepare the other ingredients.

Slice the celery, red onion and courgette on the angle. Finely chop the chilli, garlic and ginger and leave to one side.

Cook the kale in a steamer for 5 minutes. Remove and leave to one side.

Place the tofu in the roasting tin, sprinkle the sesame seeds over the tofu and roast for 15–20 minutes, until nicely caramelised.

Wash the buckwheat in a sieve and place in a pan of boiling water along with the turmeric. Cook according to the packet instructions, then drain.

Heat the oil in a frying pan, when hot add the celery, onion, courgette, chilli, garlic and ginger and fry on a high heat for 1–2 minutes, then reduce to a medium heat for 3–4 minutes until the vegetables are cooked through but still crunchy. You may need to add a tablespoon of water if the vegetables start to stick to the pan. Add the kale and tamari and cook for a further minute.

When the tofu is ready, serve with the greens and buckwheat.

Turkey escalope with sage, capers and parsley and spiced cauliflower 'couscous'

If you can only find turkey steak, there are two ways to turn it into an escalope. Depending on how thick the steak is you can either use a meat tenderiser, hammer or a rolling pin to bash the steak until it is around 5mm thick. Or, if you feel the steak is too thick for this to work, and you have a steady hand, cut the steak in half horizontally and then bash each piece with the tenderiser.

SERVES 1

150g cauliflower, roughly chopped

1 garlic clove, finely chopped

40g red onion, finely chopped

1 bird's eye chilli, finely chopped

1 tsp finely chopped fresh ginger

2 tbsp extra virgin olive oil

2 tsp ground turmeric

30g sun-dried tomatoes, finely chopped

10g parsley

150g turkey escalope or steak (see above)

1 tsp dried sage

juice of ¼ lemon

1 tbsp capers

To make the 'couscous', place the raw cauliflower in a food processor. Pulse in 2-second bursts to finely chop the cauliflower until it resembles couscous. Alternatively, you can just use a knife and chop it very finely.

Fry the garlic, red onion, chilli and ginger in 1 teaspoon of the oil until soft but not coloured. Add the turmeric and cauliflower and cook for 1 minute. Remove from the heat and add the sun-dried tomatoes and half the parsley.

Coat the turkey escalope in the sage and a little oil then fry in a frying pan set over a medium heat for 5–6 minutes, turning regularly. When cooked through, add the lemon juice, remaining parsley, capers and 1 table-spoon of water to the pan. This will create a sauce to serve with the cauliflower.

Kale and red onion dhal with buckwheat

SERVES 1

1 tsp extra virgin olive oil
1 tsp mustard seeds
40g red onion, finely chopped
1 garlic clove, finely chopped
1 tsp finely chopped fresh ginger
1 bird's eye chilli, finely chopped
1 tsp mild curry powder (medium or hot if you prefer)
2 tsp ground turmeric
300ml vegetable stock or water
40g red lentils, rinsed
50g kale, chopped
50ml tinned coconut milk
50g buckwheat

Heat the oil in a medium saucepan over a medium heat and add the mustard seeds. As the mustard seeds start to pop, add the onion, garlic, ginger and chilli. Cook for about 10 minutes, until soft.

Add the curry powder and 1 teaspoon of the turmeric and cook the spices for a couple of minutes. Add the stock and bring to the boil. Add the lentils to the pan and simmer for a further 25–30 minutes until the lentils are cooked through and you have a smooth dhal.

Add the kale and coconut milk and cook for a further 5 minutes.

Meanwhile, cook the buckwheat according to the packet instructions. Drain and serve alongside the dhal.

Aromatic chicken breast with kale and red onions and a tomato and chilli salsa

SERVES 1

120g skinless, boneless chicken breast
2 tsp ground turmeric
juice of ¼ lemon
1 tbsp extra virgin olive oil
50g kale, chopped
20g red onion, sliced
1 tsp chopped fresh ginger
50g buckwheat

For the salsa

130g tomato (about 1)
1 bird's eye chilli, finely chopped
1 tbsp capers, finely chopped
5g parsley, finely chopped
juice of ¼ lemon

To make the salsa, remove the eye from the tomato and chop it very finely, taking care to keep as much of the liquid as possible. Mix with the chilli, capers, parsley and lemon juice. You could put everything in a blender but the end result is a little different.

Heat the oven to 220°C/gas 7. Marinate the chicken breast in 1 teaspoon of the turmeric, the lemon juice and a little oil. Leave for 5–10 minutes.

Heat an ovenproof frying pan until hot, then add the marinated chicken and cook for a minute or so on each side, until pale golden, then transfer to the oven (place on a baking tray if your pan isn't ovenproof) for 8–10 minutes or until cooked through. Remove from the oven, cover with foil and leave to rest for 5 minutes before serving.

Meanwhile, cook the kale in a steamer for 5 minutes. Fry the red onions and the ginger in a little oil, until soft but not coloured, then add the cooked kale and fry for another minute.

Cook the buckwheat according to the packet instructions with the remaining teaspoon of turmeric. Serve alongside the chicken, vegetables and salsa.

Harissa baked tofu with cauliflower 'couscous'

SERVES 1

60g red pepper
1 bird's eye chilli, halved
2 garlic cloves
about 1 tbsp extra virgin olive oil
pinch of ground cumin
pinch of ground coriander
juice of ¼ lemon
200g firm tofu
200g cauliflower, roughly chopped
40g red onion, finely chopped
1 tsp finely chopped fresh ginger
2 tsp ground turmeric
30g sun-dried tomatoes, finely chopped
20g parsley, chopped

Heat the oven to 200°C/gas 6.

To make the harissa, slice the red pepper around the core so you have nice flat slices, remove any seeds then place in a roasting tin with the chilli and one of the garlic cloves. Toss with a little oil and the dried spices and roast in the oven for 15–20 minutes until the peppers are soft but not too coloured. (Leave the oven on at this setting.) Cool, then blend in a food processor with the lemon juice until smooth.

Slice the tofu lengthways and then cut each half into triangles. Place in a small non-stick roasting tin or line one with greaseproof paper, cover with the harissa and roast in the oven for 20 minutes – the tofu should have absorbed the marinade and turned a dark-red colour.

To make the 'couscous', place the raw cauliflower in a food processor. Pulse in 2-second bursts to finely chop the cauliflower until it resembles couscous. Alternatively, you can just use a knife and chop it very finely.

Finely chop the remaining garlic clove. Fry the garlic, red onion and ginger in 1 teaspoon of the oil, until soft but not coloured, then add the turmeric and cauliflower and cook for 1 minute.

Remove from the heat and stir in the sun-dried tomatoes and parsley. Serve with the baked tofu.

Sirt muesli

If you want to make this in bulk or prepare it the night before, simply combine the dry ingredients and store it in an airtight container. All you need to do the next day is add the strawberries and yoghurt and it's good to go.

SERVES 1

20g buckwheat flakes
10g buckwheat puffs
15g coconut flakes or desiccated coconut
40g Medjool dates, pitted and chopped
15g walnuts, chopped
10g cocoa nibs
100g strawberries, hulled and chopped
100g plain Greek yoghurt (or vegan alternative, such as soya or coconut yoghurt)

Mix all of the above ingredients together (leave out the strawberries and yoghurt if not serving straight away).

Pan-fried salmon fillet with caramelised chicory, rocket and celery leaf salad

SERVES 1

10g parsley
juice of ¼ lemon
1 tbsp capers
1 tbsp extra virgin olive oil
¼ avocado, peeled, stoned and diced
100g cherry tomatoes, halved
20g red onion, thinly sliced
50g rocket
5g celery leaves
150g skinless salmon fillet
2 tsp brown sugar
1 head of chicory (70g), halved lengthways

Heat the oven to 220°C/gas 7.

For the dressing, place the parsley, lemon juice, capers and 2 teaspoons of the oil in a food processor or blender and blend until smooth.

For the salad, mix the avocado, tomato, red onion, rocket and celery leaves together.

Heat an ovenproof frying pan over a high heat. Rub the salmon in a little oil and sear it in the hot pan for a minute or so to caramelise the outside of the fish. Transfer to a baking tray and return to the oven for 5–6 minutes or until cooked through; reduce the cooking time by 2 minutes if you like your fish served pink inside.

Meanwhile, wipe out the frying pan and place it back on a high heat. Mix the brown sugar with the remaining teaspoon of oil and brush it over the cut sides of the chicory. Place cut-sides down in the hot pan and cook for 2–3 minutes turning regularly, until tender and nicely caramelised all over. Toss the salad in the dressing and serve with the salmon and chicory.

Tuscan bean stew

SERVES 1

1 tbsp extra virgin olive oil
50g red onion, finely chopped
30g carrot, peeled and finely chopped
30g celery, trimmed and finely chopped
1 garlic clove, finely chopped
½ bird's eye chilli, finely chopped (optional)
1 tsp herbes de Provence
200ml vegetable stock
1 x 400g tin chopped Italian tomatoes
1 tsp tomato purée
200g tinned mixed beans
50g kale, roughly chopped
1 tbsp roughly chopped parsley
40g buckwheat

Place the oil in a medium saucepan over a low–medium heat and gently fry the onion, carrot, celery, garlic, chilli, if using, and herbs, until the onion is soft but not coloured.

Add the stock, tomatoes and tomato purée and bring to the boil. Add the beans and simmer for 30 minutes.

Add the kale and cook for another 5–10 minutes, until tender, then add the parsley.

Meanwhile, cook the buckwheat according to the packet instructions, drain and then serve with the stew.

Strawberry buckwheat tabbouleh

SERVES 1

50g buckwheat
1 tbsp ground turmeric
80g avocado
65g tomato
20g red onion
25g Medjool dates, pitted
1 tbsp capers
30g parsley
100g strawberries, hulled
1 tbsp extra virgin olive oil
juce of ½ lemon
30g rocket

Cook the buckwheat with the turmeric according to the packet instructions. Drain and keep to one side to cool.

Finely chop the avocado, tomato, red onion, dates, capers and parsley and mix with the cool buckwheat. Slice the strawberries and gently mix into the salad with the oil and lemon juice. Serve on a bed of rocket.

Miso marinated baked cod with stir-fried greens and sesame

SERVES 1

20g miso
1 tbsp mirin
1 tbsp extra virgin olive oil
200g skinless cod fillet
20g red onion, sliced
40g celery, sliced
1 garlic clove, finely chopped
1 bird's eye chilli, finely chopped
1 tsp finely chopped fresh ginger
60g green beans
50g kale, roughly chopped
1 tsp sesame seeds
5g parsley, roughly chopped
1 tbsp tamari (or soy sauce if not avoiding gluten)
30g buckwheat
1 tsp ground turmeric

Mix the miso, mirin and 1 teaspoon of the oil. Rub all over the cod and leave to marinate for 30 minutes. Heat the oven to 220°C/gas 7.

Bake the cod for 10 minutes.

Meanwhile, heat a large frying pan or wok with the remaining oil. Add the onion and stir-fry for a few minutes, then add the celery, garlic, chilli, ginger, green beans and kale. Toss and fry until the kale is tender and cooked through. You may need to add a little water to the pan to aid the cooking process.

Cook the buckwheat according to the packet instructions with the turmeric for 3 minutes.

Add the sesame seeds, parsley and tamari to the stir-fry and serve with the greens and fish.

Soba (buckwheat noodles) in a miso broth with tofu, celery and kale

SERVES 1

75g soba (buckwheat noodles)
1 tbsp extra virgin olive oil
20g red onion, sliced
1 garlic clove, finely chopped
1 tsp finely chopped ginger
300ml vegetable stock, plus a little extra if necessary
30g miso paste
50g kale, roughly chopped
50g celery, roughly chopped
1 tsp sesame seeds
100g firm tofu, cut into 0.5–1cm cubes
1 tsp tamari (optional; or soy sauce if not avoiding gluten)

Place the noodles in a pan of boiling water and cook for 5–8 minutes or aaccording to the packet instructions.

Heat the oil in a saucepan, add the onions, garlic and ginger and fry over a medium heat in the oil, until soft but not coloured. Add the stock and miso and bring to the boil.

Add the kale and celery to the miso broth and simmer gently for 5 minutes (try not to boil the miso as you will destroy the flavour and cause it to go grainy in texture). You may need to add a little more stock if it needs it.

Add the cooked noodles and sesame seeds and allow to warm through, then add the tofu. Serve in a bowl drizzled with a little tamari if wished.

Sirt super salad

SERVES 1

50g rocket
50g chicory leaves
100g smoked salmon slices
80g avocado, peeled, stoned and sliced
40g celery, sliced
20g red onion, sliced
15g walnuts, chopped
1 tbsp capers
1 large Medjool date, pitted and chopped
1 tbsp extra virgin olive oil
juice of ¼ lemon
10g parsley, chopped
10g lovage or celery leaves, chopped

Place the salad leaves on a plate or in a large bowl.

Mix all the remaining ingredients together and serve on top of the leaves.

VARIATIONS

For a **lentil** Sirt super salad, replace the smoked salmon with 100g tinned green lentils or cooked Puy lentils.

For a **chicken** Sirt super salad, replace the smoked salmon with a sliced cooked chicken breast.

For a **tuna** Sirt super salad, simply replace the smoked salmon with tinned tuna (bought in brine or oil according to preference).

Chargrilled beef with a red wine jus, onion rings, garlic kale and herb roasted potatoes

SERVES 1

100g potatoes, peeled and cut into 2cm dice
1 tbsp extra virgin olive oil
5g parsley, finely chopped
50g red onion, sliced into rings
50g kale, sliced
1 garlic clove, finely chopped
120–150g x 3.5cm-thick beef fillet steak or 2cm-thick sirloin steak
40ml red wine
150ml beef stock
1 tsp tomato purée
1 tsp cornflour, dissolved in 1 tbsp water

Heat the oven to 220°C/gas 7.

Place the potatoes in a saucepan of boiling water, bring back to the boil and cook for 4–5 minutes, then drain. Place in a roasting tin with 1 teaspoon of the oil and roast in the hot oven for 35–45 minutes. Turn the potatoes every 10 minutes to ensure even cooking. When cooked, remove from the oven, sprinkle with the chopped parsley and mix well.

Fry the onion in 1 teaspoon of the oil over a medium heat for 5–7 minutes, until soft and nicely caramelised. Keep warm.

Steam the kale for 2–3 minutes then drain. Fry the garlic gently in ½ teaspoon of oil for 1 minute, until soft but not coloured. Add the kale and fry for a further 1–2 minutes, until tender. Keep warm.

Heat an ovenproof frying pan over a high heat until smoking. Coat the meat in ½ a teaspoon of the oil and fry in the hot pan over a medium–high heat according to how you like your meat done – see our guide to the timings on page 199. If you like your meat medium it would be better to sear the meat and then transfer the pan to an oven set at 220°C/gas 7 and finish the cooking that way for the prescribed times.

Remove the meat from the pan and set aside to rest. Add the wine to the hot pan to bring up any meat residue. Bubble to reduce the wine by half, until syrupy and with a concentrated flavour.

Add the stock and tomato purée to the steak pan and bring to the boil, then add the cornflour paste to thicken your sauce, adding it a little at a time until you have your desired consistency. Stir in any of the juices from the rested steak and serve with the roasted potatoes, kale, onion rings and red wine sauce.

Steak cooking times

3.5cm-thick fillet steak

- **Blue:** about 1½ minutes each side
- **Rare:** about 2¼ minutes each side
- **Medium-rare:** about 3¼ minutes each side
- **Medium:** about 4½ minutes each side

2cm-thick sirloin steak

- **Blue:** about 1 minute each side
- **Rare:** about 1½ minutes each side
- **Medium-rare:** about 2 minutes each side
- **Medium:** about 2¼ minutes each side

Kidney bean mole with baked potato

SERVES 1

40g red onion, finely chopped
1 tsp finely chopped fresh ginger
1 garlic clove, finely chopped
1 bird's eye chilli, finely chopped
1 tsp extra virgin olive oil
1 tsp ground turmeric
1 tsp ground cumin
pinch of ground clove
pinch of ground cinnamon
1 medium baking potato
190g tinned chopped tomatoes
1 tsp brown sugar
50g red pepper, cored, seeds removed and roughly chopped
150ml vegetable stock
1 tbsp cocoa powder
1 tsp sesame seeds
2 tsp peanut butter (smooth if available, but chunky is fine)
150g tinned kidney beans
5g parsley, chopped

Heat the oven to 200°C/gas 6.

Fry the onion, ginger, garlic and chilli in the oil in a medium saucepan over a medium heat for about 10 minutes, or until soft. Add the spices and cook for a further 1–2 minutes.

Place the potato on a baking tray in the hot oven and bake for 45–60 minutes, until soft in middle (or longer depending on how crispy you like the outside).

Add the tomatoes, sugar, red pepper, stock, cocoa powder, sesame seeds, peanut butter and kidney beans and simmer gently for 45–60 minutes.

Sprinkle with the parsley to finish. Cut the potato in half and serve the mole on top.

Sirtfood omelette

SERVES 1

50g sliced streaky bacon (or 2 rashers, smoked or regular
depending on your taste)
3 medium eggs
35g red chicory, thinly sliced
5g parsley, finely chopped
1 tsp extra virgin olive oil

Heat a non-stick frying pan. Cut the bacon into thin strips
and cook over a high heat, until crispy. You do not need
to add any oil, there is enough fat in the bacon to cook
it. Remove from the pan and place on kitchen paper to
drain any excess fat. Wipe the pan clean.

Whisk the eggs and mix with the chicory and parsley.
Chop the cooked bacon into cubes and stir through
the eggs.

Heat the oil in the non-stick frying pan – the pan should
be hot but not smoking. Add the egg mixture and using
a spatula move it around the pan to start to cook the

egg. Keep the bits of cooked egg moving and swirl
the raw egg around the pan until the omelette level is
even. Reduce the heat and let the omelette firm up.
Ease the spatula around the edges and fold the
omelette in half or roll up and serve.

Baked chicken breast with walnut and parsley pesto and red onion salad

SERVES 1

15g parsley

15g walnuts

15g Parmesan cheese

1 tbsp extra virgin olive oil

juice of ½ lemon

50ml water

150g skinless chicken breast

20g red onions, finely sliced

1 tsp red wine vinegar

35g rocket

100g cherry tomatoes, halved

1 tsp balsamic vinegar

To make the pesto place the parsley, walnuts, Parmesan, olive oil, half the lemon juice and a little of the water in a food processor or blender and blend until you have a smooth paste. Add more water gradually until you have your preferred consistency.

Marinate the chicken breast in 1 tablespoon of the pesto and the remaining lemon juice in the fridge for 30 minutes; longer if possible.

Preheat the oven to 200°C/gas 6.

Heat an ovenproof frying pan over a medium–high heat. Fry the chicken in its marinade for 1 minute on either side then transfer the pan to the oven and cook for 8 minutes, or until cooked through.

Marinate the onions in the red wine vinegar for 5–10 minutes. Drain the liquid.

When the chicken is cooked, remove it from the oven, spoon another tablespoon of pesto over it and let the heat from the chicken melt the pesto. Cover with foil and leave to rest for 5 minutes before serving.

Combine the rocket, tomatoes and onion together and drizzle over the balsamic. Serve with the chicken, spooning over the remaining pesto.

Waldorf salad

SERVES 1

100g celery, roughly chopped
50g apple, roughly chopped
50g walnuts, roughly chopped
10g red onion, roughly chopped
5g parsley, chopped
1 tbsp capers
5g lovage or celery leaves, roughly chopped
1 tbsp extra virgin olive oil
1 tsp balsamic vinegar
juice of ¼ lemon
¼ tsp Dijon mustard
50g rocket
35g chicory leaves

Mix the celery, apple, walnuts and onion with the parsley, capers and lovage/celery leaves.

In a bowl, whisk the oil, vinegar, lemon juice and mustard to make the dressing.

Serve the celery mixture on top of the rocket and chicory and drizzle over the dressing.

Roasted aubergine wedges with walnut and parsley pesto and tomato salad

SERVES 1

20g parsley
20g walnuts
20g Parmesan cheese (or use a vegetarian or vegan
alternative)
1 tbsp extra virgin olive oil
juice of ¼ lemon
50ml water
1 medium aubergine (around 150g), quartered
20g red onions, sliced
5ml red wine vinegar
70g rocket
100g cherry tomatoes
5ml balsamic vinegar

Heat the oven to 200°C/gas 6.

To make the pesto place the parsley, walnuts, Parmesan, olive oil and half the lemon juice in a food processor or blender and blend until you have a smooth paste. Add the water gradually until you have the correct consistency – it should be thick enough to stick to the aubergine.

Brush the aubergine with a little of the pesto, reserving the rest to serve. Place on a baking tray and roast for 25–30 minutes, until the aubergine is golden brown, soft and moist.

Meanwhile, cover the red onion with the red wine vinegar and leave it to sit – this will soften and sweeten the onion. Drain the vinegar before serving.

Combine the rocket, tomatoes and drained onion and drizzle the balsamic vinegar over the salad. Serve with the hot aubergine, spooning the remaining pesto it.

Sirtfood smoothie

SERVES 1

100g plain Greek yoghurt or vegan alternative (soya or
coconut yoghurt)
6 walnut halves
8–10 medium strawberries, hulled
handful of kale, stalks removed
20g dark chocolate (85 per cent cocoa solids)
1 Medjool date, pitted
½ tsp ground turmeric
1–2mm slice of bird's eye chilli
200ml unsweetened almond milk

Blitz all the ingredients in a blender until smooth.

Stuffed wholemeal pitta

Wholemeal pittas are a great way to pack plenty of Sirtfoods into a quick lunch or convenient and portable packed lunch. You can play around with quantities and get creative, but ultimately all you do is load the ingredients in and it's good to go.

For a meat option

80g cooked turkey slices, chopped
20g Cheddar cheese, diced
35g cucumber, diced
30g red onion, chopped
25g rocket, chopped
10–15g walnuts, roughly chopped

For the dressing

1 tbsp extra virgin olive oil
1 tbsp balsamic vinegar
dash of lemon juice

For a vegan option

2–3 tbsp hummus
35g cucumber, diced
30g red onion, chopped
25g rocket, chopped
10-15g walnuts, roughly chopped

For the vegan dressing

1 tbsp extra virgin olive oil
dash of lemon juice

Butternut squash and date tagine with buckwheat

SERVES 4

1 tbsp extra virgin olive oil

1 red onion, finely chopped

1 tbsp finely chopped fresh ginger

3 garlic cloves, finely chopped

2 bird's eye chillies, finely chopped

1 tbsp ground cumin

1 cinnamon stick

2 tbsp ground turmeric

2 x 400g tins of chopped tomatoes

300ml vegetable stock

100g Medjool dates, pitted and chopped

1 x 400g tin of chickpeas, drained and rinsed

500g butternut squash, peeled and cut into bite-sized pieces

200g buckwheat

5g coriander, chopped

10g parsley, chopped

Heat the oven to 200°C/gas 6.

In a large casserole, fry the onion, ginger, garlic and chilli in the remaining oil for 2–3 minutes, add the cumin and cinnamon and 1 tablespoon of the turmeric and cook for a further 1–2 minutes.

Add the tomatoes, stock, dates and chickpeas and simmer gently for 45–60 minutes. You may have to add a little water from time to time to achieve a thick, sticky consistency and to make sure the pan does not run dry.

Place the squash in a roasting tin, toss with 1 tsp of oil and roast for 30 minutes until soft and charred around the edges.

Towards the end of the tagine's cooking time, cook the buckwheat according to the packet instructions with the remaining tablespoon of turmeric.

Add the roasted squash to the tagine along with the coriander and parsley and serve with the buckwheat.

Butter bean and miso dip with celery sticks and oatcakes

SERVES 4

2 x 400g tin of butter beans, drained and rinsed
3 tbsp extra virgin olive oil
2 tbsp brown miso paste
juice and grated zest of ½ unwaxed lemon
4 medium spring onions, trimmed and finely chopped
1 garlic clove, crushed
¼ bird's eye chilli, finely chopped
celery sticks, to serve
oatcakes, to serve

Simply mash all the ingredients together with a potato masher until you have a coarse mixture.

Serve as a dip with celery sticks and oatcakes.

Yoghurt with mixed berries, chopped walnuts and dark chocolate

SERVES 1

125g mixed berries
150g Greek yoghurt (or vegan alternative,
such as soya or coconut yoghurt)
25g walnuts, chopped
10g dark chocolate (85 per cent cocoa solids), grated

Simply add your preferred berries to a bowl and top
with the yoghurt.

Sprinkle with the walnuts and chocolate.

Chicken and kale curry with Bombay potatoes

SERVES 4

4 x 120–150g skinless, boneless chicken breasts, cut into bite-sized pieces

4 tbsp extra virgin olive oil

3 tbsp ground turmeric

2 red onions, sliced

2 bird's eye chillies, finely chopped

3 garlic cloves, finely chopped

1 tbsp finely chopped fresh ginger

1 tbsp mild curry powder

1 x 400g tin chopped tomatoes

500ml chicken stock

200ml coconut milk

2 cardamom pods

1 cinnamon stick

600g King Edward or Maris Piper potatoes

10g parsley, chopped

175g kale, chopped

5g coriander, chopped

Rub the chicken pieces in 1 teaspoon of the oil and
1 tablespoon of the turmeric. Leave to marinate for
30 minutes.

Fry the chicken over a high heat (there should be enough
oil in the marinade to cook the chicken) for 4–5 minutes
until nicely browned all over and cooked through, then
remove from the pan and set aside.

Heat 1 tablespoon of the oil in the frying pan over a
medium heat and add the onion, chilli, garlic and ginger.
Fry for about 10 minutes, or until soft, then add the curry
powder and another tablespoon of the turmeric and cook
for a further 1–2 minutes. Add the tomatoes to the pan,
then leave them to cook for a further 2 minutes. Add the
stock, coconut milk, cardamom and cinnamon stick and
leave to simmer for 45–60 minutes. Check the pan at
regular intervals to ensure it does not run dry – you may
have to add more stock.

Heat the oven to 220°C/gas 7. While your curry is
simmering, peel the potatoes and cut them into small
chunks. Place in boiling water with the remaining tablespoon of turmeric and boil for 5 minutes. Drain well
and allow to steam dry for a further 10 minutes. They
should be white and flaky around the edges. Transfer to
a roasting tin, toss with the remaining oil and roast for

30 minutes or until golden brown and crisp. Toss through the parsley when they're ready.

When the curry has your required consistency, add the kale, cooked chicken and coriander and cook for a further
5 minutes, to ensure the chicken is cooked through, then serve with the potatoes.

Spiced scrambled eggs

SERVES 1

1 tsp extra virgin olive oil
20g red onion, finely chopped
½ bird's eye chilli, finely chopped
3 medium eggs
50ml milk
1 tsp ground turmeric
5g parsley, finely chopped

Heat the oil in a frying pan and fry the red onion and chilli, until soft but not coloured.

Whisk together the eggs, milk, turmeric and parsley. Add to the hot pan and continue cooking over a low–medium heat, constantly moving the egg mixture around the pan to scramble it and stop it from sticking/burning. When you have achieved your desired consistency, serve.

Sirt chilli con carne

SERVES 4

1 red onion, finely chopped

3 garlic cloves, finely chopped

2 bird's eye chillies, finely chopped

1 tbsp extra virgin olive oil

1 tbsp ground cumin

1 tbsp ground turmeric

400g lean minced beef (5 per cent fat)

150ml red wine

1 red pepper, cored, seeds removed and cut into bite-sized
pieces

2 x 400g tins chopped tomatoes

1 tbsp tomato purée

1 tbsp cocoa powder

150g tinned kidney beans

300ml beef stock

5g coriander, chopped

5g parsley, chopped

160g buckwheat

In a casserole, fry the onion, garlic and chilli in the oil over a medium heat for 2–3 minutes, then add the spices and cook for a further minute or two. Add the minced beef and cook for a further 2–3 minutes over a medium–high heat until the meat is nicely browned all over. Add the red wine and allow it to bubble to reduce it by half.

Add the red pepper, tomatoes, tomato purée, cocoa, kidney beans and stock and leave to simmer for 1 hour. You may have to add a little water from time to time to achieve a thick, sticky consistency. Just before serving stir in the chopped herbs.

Meanwhile, cook the buckwheat according to the packet instructions and serve alongside the chilli.

Mushroom and tofu scramble

SERVES 1

100g extra-firm tofu
1 tsp ground turmeric
1 tsp mild curry powder
20g kale, roughly chopped
1 tsp extra virgin olive oil
20g red onion, thinly sliced
½ bird's eye chilli, thinly sliced
50g mushrooms, thinly sliced
5g parsley, finely chopped

Wrap the tofu in some kitchen paper and place something heavy on top to help it drain.

Mix the turmeric and curry powder and add a little water until you have achieved a light paste. Steam the kale for 2–3 minutes.

Heat the oil in a frying pan over a medium heat and fry the onion, chilli and mushrooms for 2–3 minutes until they have started to brown and soften.

Crumble the tofu into bite-size pieces and add to the pan, pour the spice mix over the tofu and mix thoroughly. Cook over a medium heat for 2–3 minutes so the spices are cooked through and the tofu has started to brown. Add the kale and continue to cook over a medium heat for a further minute. Finally, add the parsley, mix well and serve.

Smoked salmon pasta with chilli and rocket

SERVES 4

2 tbsp extra virgin olive oil
1 red onion, finely chopped
2 garlic cloves, finely chopped
2 bird's eye chillies, finely chopped
150g cherry tomatoes, halved
100ml white wine
250–300g buckwheat pasta
250g smoked salmon
2 tbsp capers
juice of ½ lemon
60g rocket
10g parsley, chopped

Heat 1 teaspoon of the oil in a frying pan over a medium heat. Add the onion, garlic and chilli and fry until soft but not coloured.

Add the tomatoes and leave to cook for a minute or two. Add the white wine and bubble to reduce by half.

Meanwhile, cook the pasta in boiling water with
1 teaspoon of the oil for 8–10 minutes depending on
how al dente you like it, then drain.

Slice the salmon into strips and add to the pan of tomatoes along with the capers, lemon juice, rocket and
parsley, add the pasta, mix well and serve immediately.
Drizzle any remaining oil over the top.

Buckwheat pasta salad

SERVES 1

50g buckwheat pasta, cooked according to
the packet instructions
large handful of rocket
small handful of basil leaves
8 cherry tomatoes, halved
½ avocado, diced
10 olives
1 tbsp extra virgin olive oil
20g pine nuts

Gently combine all of the ingredients except the pine
nuts and arrange on a plate, then scatter the pine nuts
over the top.

Buckwheat pancakes with strawberries, dark chocolate sauce and crushed walnuts

MAKES AROUND 6–8 PANCAKES, DEPENDING ON THE SIZE

For the pancakes

350ml milk
150g buckwheat flour
1 large egg
1 tbsp extra virgin olive oil, for cooking

For the chocolate sauce

100g dark chocolate (85 per cent cocoa solids)
85ml milk
1 tbsp double cream
1 tbsp extra virgin olive oil

To serve

400g strawberries, hulled and chopped
100g walnuts, chopped

To make the pancake batter, place all of the ingredients apart from the olive oil in a blender and blend until you have a smooth batter. It should not be too thick or too runny. (You can store any excess batter in an airtight container for up to 5 days in your fridge. Be sure to mix well before using again.)

To make the chocolate sauce, melt the chocolate in a heatproof bowl above a pan of simmering water. Once melted, mix in the milk, whisking thoroughly and then add the double cream and olive oil. You can keep the sauce warm by leaving the water in the pan simmering on a very low heat until your pancakes are ready.

To make the pancakes, heat a heavy-bottomed frying pan until it starts to smoke, then add the olive oil.

Pour some of the batter into the centre of the pan, then tip the excess batter around it until you have covered the whole surface, you may have to add a little more batter to achieve this. You will only need to cook the pancake for 1 minute or so on each side if your pan is hot enough.

Once you can see it going brown around the edges use a spatula to loosen the pancake around its edge, then flip it over. Try to flip in one action to avoid breaking it. Cook for a further minute or so on the other side and transfer to a plate.

Place some strawberries in the centre and roll up the pancake. Continue until you have made as many pancakes as required.

Spoon over a generous amount of sauce and sprinkle over some chopped walnuts.

You may find that your first efforts are too fat or fall apart but once you find the consistency for your batter that works best for you and you get your technique perfected you'll be making them like a professional. Practice makes perfect in this case.

Tofu and shiitake mushroom soup

SERVES 4

10g dried wakame
1 litre vegetable stock
200g shiitake mushrooms, sliced
120g miso paste
1 x 400g block firm tofu, cut into small cubes
2 spring onions, trimmed and sliced on the diagonal
1 bird's eye chilli, finely chopped (optional)

Soak the wakame in warm water for 10 minutes then drain.

Bring the stock to the boil, then add the mushrooms and simmer gently for 1–2 minutes.

Dissolve the miso paste in a bowl with some of the warm stock to ensure it dissolves thoroughly. Add the miso and tofu to the remaining stock, taking care not to let the soup boil as this would spoil the delicate miso flavour. Add the drained wakame, spring onions, and chilli, if using, and serve.

Sirtfood pizza

MAKES TWO 30CM PIZZAS

For the pizza base

1 x 7g packet of dried yeast
1 tsp brown sugar
300ml lukewarm water
200g buckwheat flour
200g strong white flour or tipo 00 pasta flour plus a little
extra for rolling out
1 tbsp extra virgin olive oil, plus a little extra for greasing

For the tomato sauce

½ red onion, finely chopped
1 garlic clove, finely chopped
1 tsp extra virgin olive oil
1 tsp dried oregano
2 tbsp white wine
1 x 400g tin of chopped tomatoes
pinch of brown sugar
5g basil leaves

Our favourite toppings

- Rocket, red onion and grilled aubergine (grilled auber-gine can be bought from a deli, or to grill your own, heat a griddle pan until it is starting to smoke, then reduce the heat to medium. Slice an aubergine width-ways into 3–5mm slices, brush with a little extra virgin olive oil and cook until you have achieved black grill marks on either side of the aubergine and it is nice and soft. Alternatively, you could roast the aubergine on a baking tray lined with a sheet of parchment paper at 200°C/gas 6 for 15 minutes or until soft and golden brown.)
- Chilli flakes, cherry tomato, goat's cheese and rocket
- Cooked chicken, rocket, red onion and olive
- Cooked chorizo, red onion and steamed kale

For the dough, dissolve the yeast and sugar in the water. This will help to activate the yeast. Cover with cling film and leave for 10–15 minutes.

Sift the flours into a bowl. If you have a stand mixer, fit it with the dough hook and sift the flours into the mixer bowl.

Add the yeast mixture and oil to the flour and mix together until you have formed a dough. You may have

to add a little more water if your dough is a little dry.
Knead until you have a smooth, springy dough.

Transfer the dough to an oiled bowl, cover with a clean
damp tea towel and leave somewhere warm to rise for
45–60 minutes, until doubled in size.

Meanwhile, make the tomato sauce. Fry the onion and
garlic in the olive oil until soft, then add the dried
oregano. Add the wine and bubble to reduce it by half.

Add the tomatoes and sugar, bring back to the boil and
cook for 30 minutes until the mixture is a thick consistency.
If it is too runny it will make the pizza soggy. Remove
the pan from the heat, tear the basil leaves apart with
your hands and stir them into the sauce.

Start kneading the dough again to remove the air – this
is called knocking back. After a minute or so, when you
have a nice smooth dough, it is ready. You can either use
the dough immediately or wrap it in cling film and place
in the fridge for a couple of days.

Heat the oven to 230°C/gas 8. Lightly dust a work surface
with flour. Cut the dough in half and roll out each piece
to your required thickness and place on a pizza stone or

oiled non-stick baking tray. (This quantity of dough will make two thin-crust pizzas of about 30cm in diameter. If you would like a deeper crust simply use more of the dough or reduce the size of the pizza.)

Spread a thin layer of tomato sauce over the dough (you will only need about half the sauce for this quantity of dough but freeze any left over), leaving a gap around the edge for the crust. Add the rest of your ingredients (if you're using rocket and chilli flakes, add them after you've baked your pizza). Set aside for about 15–20 minutes before baking, the dough will start to rise again giving a lighter base.

Bake in the oven for 10–12 minutes or until the cheese is golden brown. Top with rocket and chilli flakes now, if using.

Sirtfood bites

MAKES 15–20 BITES

120g walnuts
30g dark chocolate (85 per cent cocoa solids), broken into
pieces; or cocoa nibs
250g Medjool dates, pitted
1 tbsp cocoa powder
1 tbsp ground turmeric
1 tbsp extra virgin olive oil
the scraped seeds of 1 vanilla pod or 1 tsp vanilla extract
1–2 tbsp water

Place the walnuts and chocolate in a food processor and
process until you have a fine powder.

Add all the other ingredients except the water and blend
until the mixture forms a ball. You may or may not have
to add the water depending on the consistency of the
mixture – you don't want it to be too sticky.

Using your hands, form the mixture into bite-sized balls and refrigerate in an airtight container for at least 1 hour before eating them. You could roll some of the balls in some more cocoa or desiccated coconut to achieve a different finish if you like. They will keep for up to 1 week in your fridge.

Glossary

Antioxidant (dietary) A substance, either man-made or found naturally in food, which when consumed reduces the physical stress on the cells in our bodies.

Autophagy The process by which our cells break down and recycle waste material and debris in order to use it for fuel. Autophagy is increased during periods of cellular stress.

Blue Zones Select geographical regions of the world where people eat diets rich in Sirtfoods and live extraordinarily long, healthy, and happy lives.

Caloric restriction A dietary regimen where people purposely reduce their food intake in an attempt to lose weight, improve health and extend lifespan.

Circadian rhythm Our natural body clock that runs on a 24-hour cycle and regulates the activity and efficiency of many important physiological processes, such as sleep and how we process food, according to the time of the day.

DHA (Docosahexaenoic acid) One of two crucial omega-3 fatty acids (alongside EPA), primarily found in oily fish and marine plants like algae, which enhances the activity of our sirtuins and improves overall health.

EPA (Eicosapentaenoic acid) One of two crucial omega-3 fatty acids (alongside DHA), primarily found in oily fish, which enhances the activity of our sirtuins and improves overall health.

Gene Made up of DNA, the blueprint of our body; when activated a gene signals our bodies to produce protein which changes how our cells work.

Hormesis A biological phenomenon whereby exposure to something that is bad for us in high amounts is actually beneficial in small and moderate quantities. Examples include exercise and fasting.

Inflammaging A persistent, low-grade inflammation that occurs with aging and increases our risk of many chronic diseases.

Intermittent fasting An umbrella term for any diet that is characterised by alternating periods of caloric restriction (fasting days) and ad lib feeding. Fasting days are usually limited to between 1 and 3 days a week and so usually more intense than normal caloric restriction.

Leucine An essential amino acid found in dietary protein. It has a potent effect in enhancing the benefits of Sirtfoods, so a Sirtfood diet should also be protein-rich.

Master Regulator A gene or something that influences a gene, that is at the top of a hierarchy that regulates and controls other genes below it.

Metabolism All of the biochemical reactions taking place within a cell that help maintain life.

Mitochondria Tiny structures within a cell that break down nutrients and generate energy. They power the cell to carry out its functions. Muscle cells require a lot of energy so are particularly rich in mitochondria.

mTOR (mammalian target of rapamycin) A vital growth promotor in the body, but its activity needs to be kept in check or else disease can occur. Its activity is highly influenced by the food we eat.

Muscle Gain Adjusted Weight Loss A method for calculating weight loss where reported weight loss results are not penalised for a desirable increase in muscle. This is a much more accurate way of reflecting changes to overall body composition than simply weight loss alone.

PGC1 alpha (Peroxisome proliferator-activated receptor-gamma coactivator 1 alpha) A key regulator of energy metabolism that stimulates the creation of mitochondria in our cells (see Mitochondria above).

Polyphenols A vast group of natural chemicals found in plants that are part of a plants defences against environmental stresses. Certain polyphenols switch on our sirtuin genes, when consumed, and give rise to the many benefits of the Sirtfood Diet.

PPAR-ɣ (peroxisome proliferator-activated receptor-ɣ) A key regulator of metabolism in our cells that switches on genes involved in synthesising and storing fat.

Sirt-1 The most thoroughly researched of the sirtuin family of genes and the most important for targeting weight loss. It is activated when cells are stressed, and has numerous health and anti-ageing effects.

Sirtfood A food particularly rich in specific polyphenols that, when we consume them, are able to activate our sirtuin genes.

Sirtuin An ancient family of genes that exist in all of us that are activated when our cells are put under stress. Sirtuins play an important role in health, disease prevention and ageing. In humans, there are seven different sirtuins (Sirt-1 to Sirt-7). Of these Sirt-1 and Sirt-3 are the two most important sirtuins involved in energy balance.

Stem cell A special type of cell that can grow into any type of cell found in the body.

Western diet The typical diet representative of industrialised, modern eating patterns, and the antithesis of the Blue Zones. A Western diet is characterised by a high consumption of processed and refined foods and a notable lack of nutrient-rich plants, especially Sirtfoods.

Xenohormesis The biological phenomenon whereby humans can piggyback on the stress responses of plants and experience a wealth of benefits by consuming the polyphenols they produce.

References

Introduction

1. Hill, A.J. 'Does dieting make you fat?' *Br J Nutr* **92** Suppl 1, S15–18 (2004).
2. Harvie, M.N. et al. 'The effects of intermittent or continuous energy restriction on weight loss and metabolic disease risk markers: a randomized trial in young overweight women.' *Int J Obes (Lond)* **35**, 714–27 (2011).
3. Howitz, K.T. et al. 'Small molecule activators of sirtuins extend Saccharomyces cerevisiae lifespan.' *Nature* **425**, 191–6 (2003).
4. Wang, L., Lee, I.M., Manson, J.E., Buring, J.E. & Sesso, H.D. 'Alcohol consumption, weight gain, and risk of becoming overweight in middle-aged and older women.' *Arch Intern Med* **170**, 453–61 (2010).
5. Malhotra, A., 'Maruthappu, M. & Stephenson, T. 'Healthy eating: an NHS priority A sure way to improve health

outcomes for NHS staff and the public.' *Postgrad Med J* **90**, 671–2 (2014).

6. Agudelo, L.Z. et al. 'Skeletal muscle PGC-1alpha1 modulates kynurenine metabolism and mediates resilience to stress-induced depression.' *Cell* **159**, 33–45 (2014).

Chapter 1 The Science of Sirtuins

7. Li, X. 'SIRT1 and energy metabolism.' *Acta Biochim Biophys Sin* (Shanghai) **45**, 51–60 (2013).

8. Morris, B.J. 'Seven sirtuins for seven deadly diseases of aging.' *Free Radic Biol Med* **56**, 133–71 (2013).

9. Fontana, L., Partridge, L. & Longo, V.D. 'Extending healthy life span–from yeast to humans.' *Science* **328**, 321–6 (2010).

10. Ibid.

11. Haigis, M.C. & Guarente, L.P. 'Mammalian sirtuins– emerging roles in physiology, aging, and calorie restriction.' *Genes Dev* **20**, 2913–21 (2006).

12. Radak, Z. et al. 'Redox-regulating sirtuins in aging, caloric restriction, and exercise.' *Free Radic Biol Med* **58**, 87–97 (2013).

13. Selinger, J.C., O'Connor, S.M., Wong, J.D. & Donelan, J.M. 'Humans Can Continuously Optimize Energetic Cost during Walking.' *Curr Biol* **25**, 2452–6 (2015).

14. Schnohr, P., O'Keefe, J.H., Marott, J.L., Lange, P. & Jensen, G.B. 'Dose of jogging and long-term mortality: the Copenhagen City Heart Study.' *J Am Coll Cardiol* **65**, 411–9 (2015).

15. Mons, U., Hahmann, H. & Brenner, H. 'A reverse J-shaped association of leisure time physical activity with prognosis

in patients with stable coronary heart disease: evidence from a large cohort with repeated measurements.' *Heart* **100**, 1043–9 (2014).

Chapter 2 Fighting Fat

16. Bordone, L. et al. 'SIRT1 transgenic mice show phenotypes resembling calorie restriction.' *Aging Cell* **6**, 759–67 (2007).

17. Chalkiadaki, A. & Guarente, L. 'High-fat diet triggers inflammation-induced cleavage of SIRT1 in adipose tissue to promote metabolic dysfunction.' *Cell Metab* **16**, 180-8 (2012).

18. Costa Cdos, S. et al. 'SIRT1 transcription is decreased in visceral adipose tissue of morbidly obese patients with severe hepatic steatosis.' *Obes Surg* **20**, 633–9 (2010).

19. Pedersen, S.B., Olholm, J., Paulsen, S.K., Bennetzen, M.F. & Richelsen, B. 'Low Sirt1 expression, which is upregulated by fasting, in human adipose tissue from obese women.' *Int J Obes* (Lond) **32**, 1250–5 (2008).

20. Zillikens, M.C. et al. 'SIRT1 genetic variation is related to BMI and risk of obesity.' *Diabetes* **58**, 2828–34 (2009).

21. Tontonoz, P. & Spiegelman, B.M. 'Fat and beyond: the diverse biology of PPARgamma.' *Annu Rev Biochem* **77**, 289–312 (2008).

22. Picard, F. et al. 'Sirt1 promotes fat mobilization in white adipocytes by repressing PPAR-gamma.' *Nature* **429**, 771–6 (2004).

23. Qiang, L. et al. 'Brown remodeling of white adipose tissue by SirT1-dependent deacetylation of Ppargamma.' *Cell* **150**, 620–32 (2012).

24. Li, X. 'SIRT1 and energy metabolism.' *Acta Biochim Biophys Sin* (Shanghai) **45**, 51–60 (2013).

25. Akieda-Asai, S. et al. 'SIRT1 Regulates Thyroid-Stimulating Hormone Release by Enhancing PIP5Kgamma Activity through Deacetylation of Specific Lysine Residues in Mammals.' *PLoS One* **5**, e11755 (2010).

26. Sasaki, T. et al. 'Induction of hypothalamic Sirt1 leads to cessation of feeding via agouti-related peptide.' *Endocrinology* **151**, 2556–66 (2010).

27. Sasaki, T. et al. 'Hypothalamic SIRT1 prevents age-associated weight gain by improving leptin sensitivity in mice.' *Diabetologia* **57**, 819–31 (2014).

Chapter 3 Masters of Muscle

28. Sharples, A.P. et al. 'Longevity and skeletal muscle mass: the role of IGF signalling, the sirtuins, dietary restriction and protein intake.' *Aging Cell* **14**, 511–23 (2015).

29. Diaz-Ruiz, A., Gonzalez-Freire, M., Ferrucci, L., Bernier, M. & de Cabo, R. 'SIRT1 synchs satellite cell metabolism with stem cell fate.' *Cell Stem Cell* **16**, 103–4 (2015).

30. Rathbone, C.R., Booth, F.W. & Lees, S.J. 'Sirt1 increases skeletal muscle precursor cell proliferation.' *Eur J Cell Biol* **88**, 35–44 (2009).

31. Lee, D. & Goldberg, A.L. 'SIRT1 protein, by blocking the activities of transcription factors FoxO1 and FoxO3, inhibits muscle atrophy and promotes muscle growth.' *J Biol Chem* **288**, 30515–26 (2013).

32. Ryall, J.G. et al. 'The NAD(+)-dependent SIRT1 deacetylase translates a metabolic switch into regulatory epigenetics in skeletal muscle stem cells.' *Cell Stem Cell* **16**, 171–83 (2015).

33. Lee & Goldberg, 'SIRT1 protein'.

34. Sharples, 'Longevity and skeletal muscle mass'.

35. Lee & Goldberg, 'SIRT1 protein'.

36. Ibid.

37. Sharples, 'Longevity and skeletal muscle mass'.

38. Sousa-Victor, P., García-Prat, L., Serrano, A.L., Perdiguero, E. & Muñoz-Cánoves, P. 'Muscle stem cell aging: regulation and rejuvenation.' *Trends Endocrinol Metab* **26**, 287–96 (2015).

39. Tonkin, J., Villarroya, F., Puri, P.L. & Vinciguerra, M. 'SIRT1 signaling as potential modulator of skeletal muscle diseases.' *Curr Opin Pharmacol* **12**, 372–6 (2012).

40. Cohen, S., Nathan, J.A. & Goldberg, A.L. 'Muscle wasting in disease: molecular mechanisms and promising therapies.' *Nat Rev Drug Discov* **14**, 58–74 (2015).

Chapter 4 Well-being Wonders

41. Ma, L. & Li, Y. 'SIRT1: role in cardiovascular biology.' *Clin Chim Acta* **440**, 8–15 (2015).

42. Ibid.

43. Milne, J.C. et al. 'Small molecule activators of SIRT1 as therapeutics for the treatment of type 2 diabetes.' *Nature* **450**, 712–6 (2007).

44. Fu, L. et al. 'Leucine amplifies the effects of metformin on

insulin sensitivity and glycemic control in diet-induced obese mice.' *Metabolism* **64**, 845–56 (2015).

45. Wang, J. et al. 'The role of Sirt1: at the crossroad between promotion of longevity and protection against Alzheimer's disease neuropathology.' *Biochim Biophys Acta* **1804**, 1690–4 (2010).

46. Giblin, W., Skinner, M.E. & Lombard, D.B. 'Sirtuins: guardians of mammalian healthspan.' *Trends Genet* **30**, 271–86 (2014).

47. Iyer, S. et al. 'Sirtuin1 (Sirt1) promotes cortical bone formation by preventing beta-catenin sequestration by FoxO transcription factors in osteoblast progenitors.' *J Biol Chem* **289**, 24069–78 (2014).

48. Wilking, M.J. & Ahmad, N. 'The role of SIRT1 in cancer: the saga continues.' *Am J Pathol* **185**, 26–8 (2015).

Chapter 5 Sirtfoods

49. Leitzmann, M.F. et al. 'Physical activity recommendations and decreased risk of mortality.' *Arch Intern Med* **167**, 2453–60 (2007).

50. Kennedy, D.O. 'Polyphenols and the human brain: plant "secondary metabolite" ecologic roles and endogenous signaling functions drive benefits.' *Adv Nutr* **5**, 515–33 (2014).

51. Hooper, P.L., Hooper, P.L., Tytell, M. & Vigh, L. 'Xenohormesis: health benefits from an eon of plant stress

response evolution.' *Cell Stress Chaperones* **15**, 761–70 (2010).

52. Ibid.

53. Howitz, K.T. & Sinclair, D.A. 'Xenohormesis: sensing the chemical cues of other species.' *Cell* **133**, 387–91 (2008).

54. Howitz, K.T. et al. 'Small molecule activators of sirtuins extend Saccharomyces cerevisiae lifespan.' *Nature* **425**, 191–6 (2003).

55. Madeo, F., Pietrocola, F., Eisenberg, T. & Kroemer, G. 'Caloric restriction mimetics: towards a molecular definition.' *Nat Rev Drug Discov* **13**, 727–40 (2014).

Chapter 6 Sirtfoods Around the World

56. Bayard, V., Chamorro, F., Motta, J. & Hollenberg, N.K. 'Does flavanol intake influence mortality from nitric oxide-dependent processes? Ischemic heart disease, stroke, diabetes mellitus, and cancer in Panama.' *Int J Med Sci* **4**, 53–8 (2007).

57. Shrime, M.G. et al. 'Flavonoid-rich cocoa consumption affects multiple cardiovascular risk factors in a meta-analysis of short-term studies.' *J Nutr* **141**, 1982–8 (2011).

58. Hooper, L. et al. 'Effects of chocolate, cocoa, and flavan-3-ols on cardiovascular health: a systematic review and meta-analysis of randomized trials.' *Am J Clin Nutr* **95**, 740–51 (2012).

59. Duarte, D.A. et al. 'Polyphenol-enriched cocoa protects the

diabetic retina from glial reaction through the sirtuin pathway.' *J Nutr Biochem* **26**, 64–74 (2015).

60. Martin, M.A., Goya, L. & Ramos S. 'Potential for preventive effects of cocoa and cocoa polyphenols in cancer.' *Food Chem Toxicol* **56**, 336-51 (2013).

61. Brickman, A.M. et al. 'Enhancing dentate gyrus function with dietary flavanols improves cognition in older adults.' *Nat Neurosci* **17**, 1798–803 (2014).

62. Hutchins-Wolfbrandt, A. & Mistry, A.M. 'Dietary turmeric potentially reduces the risk of cancer.' *Asian Pac J Cancer Prev* **12**, 3169–73 (2011).

63. Panahi, Y. et al. 'Antioxidant and anti-inflammatory effects of curcuminoid-piperine combination in subjects with metabolic syndrome: A randomized controlled trial and an updated meta-analysis.' *Clin Nutr* (2015).

64. Kuptniratsaikul, V., Thanakhumtorn, S., Chinswangwatanakul, P., Wattanamongkonsil, L. & Thamlikitkul, V. 'Efficacy and safety of Curcuma domestica extracts in patients with knee osteoarthritis.' *J Altern Complement Med* **15**, 891–7 (2009).

65. Lee, M.S. et al. 'Turmeric improves post-prandial working memory in pre-diabetes independent of insulin.' *Asia Pac J Clin Nutr* **23**, 581–91 (2014).

66. Sofi, F., Cesari, F., Abbate, R., Gensini, G.F. & Casini, A. 'Adherence to Mediterranean diet and health status: meta-analysis.' *BMJ* **11**, 337:a1344 (2008).

67. Estruch, R. et al. 'Primary prevention of cardiovascular disease with a Mediterranean diet.' *N Engl J Med* **368**, 1279–90 (2013).

68. Salas-Salvado, J. et al. 'Prevention of diabetes with Mediterranean diets: a subgroup analysis of a randomized trial.' *Ann Intern Med* **160**, 1–10 (2014).

69. Estruch, R. 'Anti-inflammatory effects of the Mediterranean diet: the experience of the PREDIMED study.' *Proc Nutr Soc* **69**, 333–40 (2010).

70. Valls-Pedret, C. et al. 'Mediterranean Diet and Age-Related Cognitive Decline: A Randomized Clinical Trial.' *JAMA Intern Med* **175**, 1094–103 (2015).

71. Razquin, C. et al. 'The Mediterranean diet protects against waist circumference enlargement in 12Ala carriers for the PPARgamma gene: 2 years' follow-up of 774 subjects at high cardiovascular risk.' *Br J Nutr* **102**, 672–9 (2009).

72. Ibarrola-Jurado, N. et al. 'Cross-sectional assessment of nut consumption and obesity, metabolic syndrome and other cardiometabolic risk factors: the PREDIMED study.' *PLoS One* **8**, e57367 (2013).

Chapter 7 The Sirtfood Diet

73. Hertog, M.G. et al. 'Flavonoid intake and long-term risk of coronary heart disease and cancer in the seven countries study.' *Arch Intern Med* **155**, 381–6 (1995).

74. Ibid.

75. Biagi, M. & Bertelli, A.A. 'Wine, alcohol and pills: What future for the French paradox?' *Life Sci* **131**, 19–22 (2015).

76. Ortuño, J. et al. 'Matrix effects on the bioavailability of resveratrol in humans.' *Food Chemistry* **120**, 1123–1130 (2010).

77. Eseberri, I., Miranda, J., Lasa, A., Churruca, I. & Portillo, M.P. 'Doses of Quercetin in the Range of Serum Concentrations Exert Delipidating Effects in 3T3-L1 Preadipocytes by Acting on Different Stages of Adipogenesis, but Not in Mature Adipocytes.' *Oxid Med Cell Longev* **2015**, 480943 (2015).

78. Scheepens, A., Tan, K. & Paxton, J.W. 'Improving the oral bioavailability of beneficial polyphenols through designed synergies.' *Genes Nutr* **5**, 75–87 (2010).

79. Bohn, T. 'Dietary factors affecting polyphenol bioavailability.' *Nutr Rev* **72**, 429–52 (2014).

80. Yu, Y. et al. 'Green tea catechins: a fresh flavor to anticancer therapy.' *Apoptosis* **19**, 1–18 (2014).

81. Bruckbauer, A. & Zemel, M.B. 'Synergistic effects of polyphenols and methylxanthines with Leucine on AMPK/Sirtuin-mediated metabolism in muscle cells and adipocytes.' *PLoS One* **9**, e89166 (2014).

82. Bruckbauer, A. & Zemel, M.B. 'Effects of dairy consumption on SIRT1 and mitochondrial biogenesis in adipocytes and muscle cells.' *Nutr Metab (Lond)* **8**, 91 (2011).

83. Feldman, J.L., Baeza, J. & Denu, J.M. 'Activation of the protein deacetylase SIRT6 by long-chain fatty acids and widespread deacylation by mammalian sirtuins.' *J Biol Chem* **288**, 31350–6 (2013).

84. Wegner, D.M., Schneider, D.J., Carter, S.R. 3rd & White, T.L. 'Paradoxical effects of thought suppression.' *J Pers Soc Psychol* **53**, 5–13 (1987).

Chapter 8 Phase 1: 7lb in Seven Days

85. Bohn, T. 'Dietary factors affecting polyphenol bioavailability.' *Nutr Rev* **72**, 429–52 (2014).

86. Quinones, M., Al-Massadi, O., Ferno, J. & Nogueiras, R. 'Cross-talk between SIRT1 and endocrine factors: effects on energy homeostasis.' *Mol Cell Endocrinol* **397**, 42–50 (2014).

87. Duarte, G.S. & Farah, A. 'Effect of simultaneous consumption of milk and coffee on chlorogenic acids' bioavailability in humans.' *J Agric Food Chem* **59**, 7925–31 (2011).

88. Hursel, R. & Westerterp-Plantenga, M.S. 'Consumption of milk-protein combined with green tea modulates diet-induced thermogenesis.' *Nutrients* **3**, 725–33 (2011).

89. Green, R.J., Murphy, A.S., Schulz, B., Watkins, B.A. & Ferruzzi, M.G. 'Common tea formulations modulate in vitro digestive recovery of green tea catechins.' *Mol Nutr Food Res* **51**, 1152–62 (2007).

90. Crozier, A., Lean, M.E., McDonald, M.S. & Black, C. 'Quantitative analysis of the flavonoid content of commercial tomatoes, onions, lettuce, and celery.' *Journal of Agricultural and Food Chemistry* **45**, 590–595 (1997).

91. Bastian, B., Jetten, J. & Ferris, L.J. 'Pain as social glue: shared pain increases cooperation.' *Psychol Sci* **25**, 2079–85 (2014).

92. Lv, J. et al. 'Consumption of spicy foods and total and cause specific mortality: population based cohort study.' *BMJ* **351**, h3942 (2015).

93. Ding, M., Bhupathiraju, S.N., Chen, M., van Dam, R.M. & Hu, F.B. 'Caffeinated and decaffeinated coffee consumption and risk of type 2 diabetes: a systematic review and a dose-response meta-analysis.' *Diabetes Care* **37**, 569–86 (2014).

94. Bohn, S.K., Blomhoff, R. & Paur, I. 'Coffee and cancer risk, epidemiological evidence, and molecular mechanisms.' *Mol Nutr Food Res* **58**, 915–30 (2014).

95. Wirdefeldt, K., Adami, H.O., Cole, P., Trichopoulos, D. & Mandel, J. 'Epidemiology and etiology of Parkinson's disease: a review of the evidence.' *Eur J Epidemiol* **26 Suppl 1**, S1–58 (2011).

96. Masterton, G.S. & Hayes, P.C. 'Coffee and the liver: a potential treatment for liver disease?' *Eur J Gastroenterol Hepatol* **22**, 1277–83 (2010).

97. Alkaabi, J.M. et al. 'Glycemic indices of five varieties of dates in healthy and diabetic subjects.' *Nutr J* **10**, 59 (2011).

99. Vayalil, P.K. 'Date fruits (Phoenix dactylifera Linn): an emerging medicinal food.' *Crit Rev Food Sci Nutr* **52**, 249–71 (2012).

99. Baliga, M.S., Baliga, B.R.V., Kandathil, S.M., Bhat, H.P. & Vayalil, P.K. 'A review of the chemistry and pharmacology of the date fruits (Phoenix dactylifera L.).' *Food Research International* **44**, 1812–1822 (2011).

100. Torronen, R. et al. 'Berries reduce postprandial insulin responses to wheat and rye breads in healthy women.' *J Nutr* **143**, 430–6 (2013).

Chapter 9 Phase 2: Maintenance

101. Antunes, L.C., Levandovski, R., Dantas, G., Caumo, W. & Hidalgo, M.P. 'Obesity and shift work: chronobiological aspects.' *Nutr Res Rev* **23**, 155–68 (2010).
102. Pan, A., Schernhammer, E.S., Sun, Q. & Hu, F.B. 'Rotating night shift work and risk of type 2 diabetes: two prospective cohort studies in women.' *PLoS Med* **8**, e1001141 (2011).

Chapter 10 Sirtfoods for Life

103. Melnik, B.C. 'Milk—A Nutrient System of Mammalian Evolution Promoting mTORC1-Dependent Translation.' *International Journal of Molecular Sciences* **16**, 17048–17087 (2015).
104. Liu, M. et al. 'Resveratrol inhibits mTOR signaling by promoting the interaction between mTOR and DEPTOR'. *J Biol Chem* **285**, 36387–94 (2010).
105. Aune, D. et al. Dairy products and colorectal cancer risk: a systematic review and meta-analysis of cohort studies. *Ann Oncol* **23**, 37–45 (2012).
106. Aune, D. et al. Dairy products, calcium, and prostate cancer risk: a systematic review and meta-analysis of cohort studies. *Am J Clin Nutr* **101**, 87–117 (2015).
107. Davoodi, H., Esmaeili, S. & Mortazavian, A. 'Effects of milk and milk products consumption on cancer: A Review.'

Comprehensive Reviews in Food Science and Food Safety **12**, 249–264 (2013).

108. Wiseman, M. 'The second World Cancer Research Fund/ American Institute for Cancer Research expert report. Food, nutrition, physical activity, and the prevention of cancer: a global perspective.' *Proc Nutr Soc* **67**, 253–6 (2008).

109. Persson, E., Graziani, G., Ferracane, R., Fogliano, V. & Skog, K. 'Influence of antioxidants in virgin olive oil on the formation of heterocyclic amines in fried beefburgers.' *Food Chem Toxicol* **41**, 1587–97 (2003).

110. Gibis, M. Effect of oil marinades with garlic, onion, and lemon juice on the formation of heterocyclic aromatic amines in fried beef patties. *J Agric Food Chem* **55**, 10240–7 (2007).

111. Rohrmann, S., Hermann, S. & Linseisen, J. 'Heterocyclic aromatic amine intake increases colorectal adenoma risk: findings from a prospective European cohort study.' *Am J Clin Nutr* **89**, 1418–24 (2009).

112. Nerurkar, P.V., Le Marchand, L. & Cooney, R.V. 'Effects of marinating with Asian marinades or western barbecue sauce on PhIP and MeIQx formation in barbecued beef.' *Nutr Cancer* **34**, 147–52 (1999).

113. Rong, Y. et al. 'Egg consumption and risk of coronary heart disease and stroke: dose-response meta-analysis of prospective cohort studies.' *BMJ* **346**, e8539 (2013).

114. Duffield-Lillico, A.J. et al. 'Selenium supplementation, baseline plasma selenium status and incidence of prostate cancer: an analysis of the complete treatment period of

the Nutritional Prevention of Cancer Trial.' *BJU Int* **91**, 608–12 (2003).

115. Rayman, M.P. 'Food-chain selenium and human health: emphasis on intake.' *Br J Nutr* **100**, 254–68 (2008).

116. Ibid.

117. Craig, W.J., Mangels, A.R. & American Dietetic Association. 'Position of the American Dietetic Association: vegetarian diets.' *J Am Diet Assoc* **109**, 1266–82 (2009).

118. Appleby, P., Roddam, A., Allen, N. & Key, T. 'Comparative fracture risk in vegetarians and nonvegetarians in EPIC-Oxford.' *Eur J Clin Nutr* **61**, 1400–6 (2007).

119. Krajcovicova-Kudlackova, M., Buckova, K., Klimes, I. & Sebokova, E. 'Iodine deficiency in vegetarians and vegans.' *Ann Nutr Metab* **47**, 183–5 (2003).

Index

Acknowledgements

We would like to thank Public Health Expert Dr Padhraig Ryan of Trinity College Dublin for his invaluable input to the design of the study and analysis and reporting of outcomes.

A huge thanks to the brilliant chef Mark McCulloch for the recipes that grace this book, which prove beyond doubt that healthy eating and delicious-tasting food are not mutually exclusive.

We extend our gratitude to Gideon Remfry, and everyone at KX, not just for listening to our ideas, but for allowing the seeds of our ideas to flourish and grow. We truly hope that the publication of this book will spur much-needed future research in this exciting field.

Our thanks too to Eugenie Furniss and Rory Scarfe at Furniss Lawton, who grasped the life-changing potential of our ideas in an instant and have supported us every step of the way into making this book a reality.

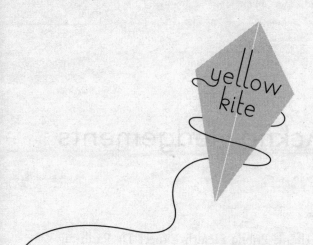

books to help you live a good life

Join the conversation and tell
us how you live a #goodlife

🐦 @yellowkitebooks
📘 YellowKiteBooks
📌 Yellow Kite Books
📷 YellowKiteBooks